Praise for Every Woman's BirthRights

"Don't write your birth plan before reading Every Woman's BirthRights. Here is a book that demystifies the birth process – from decoding pregnancy case notes, to understanding the implications of diagnostic testing, avoiding a mis-managed labour and breaking the post-natal conspiracy of silence.

"Pat Thomas takes us behind the scenes to find out what makes health professionals tick and how to get the most out of them. Her work will help restore the continued imbalance between the birthing woman and those whose job it is to support her."

Deborah Jackson, author of *Three in a Bed – Why you should sleep with your baby* and *Do Not Disturb – The benefits of relaxed parenting.*

"A marvellous antidote to the misinformed pap served up by most pregnancy and birth manuals. Pat Thomas' meticulous research exposes as empty and unscientific much of the usual advice doled out to pregnant women by the 'experts'. The moment you have a positive pregnancy test, *Every Woman's Birthrights* should be your ante-natal 'bible'."

Lynne McTaggart, Editor, *What Doctors Don't Tell You* and *Mothers Know Best*

"All too often, the information about maternity care which is given to women by health professionals is biased, incomplete and even inaccurate. This is why this book is so important. It is an unbiased presentation of the facts from a woman's perspective. At the same time, all the information here is based on the latest evidence and presented in an easily understood form. I would recommend every pregnant woman to buy, read and then use *Every Woman's BirthRights* as a continuing source of information throughout her reproductive years."

Dr Marsden Wagner, World Health Organisation; author of *Pursuing The Birth Machine – The search for appropriate birth technology.*

"Without any effort, the readers of *Every Woman's BirthRights* will absorb the content of a serious, updated and commented childbearing encyclopaedia."

Dr Michel Odent, natural childbirth pioneer; Head of Research, The Primal Health Research Centre; author of *Birth Reborn, Primal Health* and *The Nature of Birth and Breastfeeding.*

"This book spells out in clear, sometimes amusing, and forthright terms, the kind of information most women need and few women get...essential reading for every pregnant and labouring woman."

Beverley A. Lawrence Beech, Hon, Chair, Association for Improvements in the Maternity Services (AIMS); Member of the Midwifery Committee of the United Kingdom Central Council for Nurses, Midwives and Health Visitors (UKCC); author of *Who's Having Your Baby?* and co-author of *Ultrasound, Unsound?*

"A very interesting addition to the literature available. It empowers parents to know their rights and suggests practical ways of ensuring that they understand the healthcare system operational in the United Kingdom."

Yehudi Gordon, Consultant Obstetrician and co-author of *The Encyclopaedia of Pregnancy and Birth.*

Every Woman's BirthRights

Pat Thomas

Thorsons
An Imprint of HarperCollins*Publishers*

This book is dedicated to my late father, J. W. Shows, whose support, enthusiasm and faith continue to sustain me; and to my son, Alexander, without whom it might never have been written.

Thorsons
An Imprint of HarperCollins*Publishers*
77–85 Fulham Palace Road,
Hammersmith, London W6 8JB
1160 Battery Street,
San Francisco, California 94111–1213

Published by Thorsons 1996
10 9 8 7 6 5 4 3 2 1

© Pat Thomas 1996

Pat Thomas asserts the moral right to
be identified as the author of this work

A catalogue record for this book
is available from the British Library

ISBN 0 7225 3281 4

Printed and bound in Great Britain by
Caledonian International Book Manufacturing Ltd, Glasgow

All rights reserved. No part of this publication may be
reproduced, stored in a retrieval system, or transmitted,
in any form or by any means, electronic, mechanical,
photocopying, recording or otherwise, without the prior
permission of the publishers.

Contents

Acknowledgements vii
Introduction ix

Chapter One: Looking Ahead – Birth Options 1
   Hospital Care 3
   When Can You Leave? 10
   What Can You Eat? 13
   Home Birth 15
   Who Should Be There? 22
   Giving Birth in Different Positions 27
   Water Labour, Water Birth 34
   For the Baby's Good? 38

Chapter Two: Meeting the 'Experts' 43
   Mothers and Doctors 45
   General Practitioners 49
   Midwives 53
   Obstetricians 60
   Health Visitors 65

Paediatricians 67
  Students 69
  Good Practitioners and Good Patients 72

Chapter Three: The Ante-natal Routine 77
  So What Are They Looking For? 78
  The Baby's Well-being 82
  The Mother's Well-being 92
  Lifestyle 101
  General Issues in Ante-natal Care 108
  Medical Language 121

Chapter Four: Testing, Testing 125
  Routine Screening 126
  Diagnostic Tests 141
  Getting Off the Conveyor Belt 157

Chapter Five: Managing Labour 161
  Speeding Labour Up 164
  Monitoring 177
  Pain 186
  Assisting Labour 201
  The Third Stage of Labour 218

Chapter Six: Back to Normal? 223

Appendix A: Complaining About Care 235
Appendix B: Maternity Rights and Benefits 243
Appendix C: Support and Information 261

References 275
Index 291

Acknowledgements

Writing a book is something like giving birth – there are moments of enthusiasm, panic, self-doubt and triumph (I am very grateful to Caroline Flint for pointing this out to me a long time ago). This book had many midwives. Thanks to Laura Longrigg for believing in me and working so hard on my behalf. Heartfelt gratitude to Alice Charlwood, Sandar Warshal, Beverley Lawrence Beech, Christine Grabowska and Nadine Edwards, all of whom took time out from their eternally busy schedules to read the early drafts of this book and supply criticism and encouragement in equal measure. Thanks to Lynne McTaggart and Bryan Hubbard at What Doctors Don't Tell You for simpatico. Also to Joel Ryce and Jennifer Forssander for care and feeding of my psyche during its dark journeys. Warm appreciation and love to Tessa Rome for beer and flowers when my spirits were flagging, and to Bob Suter for PC guidance. I am grateful to everyone at the MIDIRS Database, especially John Loy, for the speed and efficiency with which they met my incessant, hungry requests for more information. Also to everyone at Thorsons, in particular Erica Smith for her faith and editorial judgement and Barbara Vesey for her thoughtful copy editing.

No progress could have been made on the manuscript without the help of other women who were prepared to entertain, care for and generally 'mother' my son while I worked. For her generosity and flexibility, my gratitude and thanks go out particularly to Arlene Neckles and her family. Finally I would like to thank my son, Alexander, who displayed forbearance, love and an awareness of the importance of the task, above and beyond his four years, when I was obliged to play with the computer instead of him. I love you very much. Also to everyone at Thorsons, in particular Erica Smith for her faith and editorial judgement and Barbara Vesey for her thoughtful copy editing.

Introduction

It could be argued that the ability to make choices is one of the most important skills a new mother can have. It is a skill which she will exercise again and again in her role as a parent. From the moment pregnancy is confirmed, women are confronted by a staggering range of choices and decisions. Even the smallest of these is often made against the complex backdrop of practical, material, emotional, physical, cultural and religious factors which mothers negotiate daily in order to get the best for themselves and their families.

What's more, some of the most difficult decisions a mother can make today confront her before her baby is even born. It is all too easy for women to be romanced into believing that a carefree pregnancy and ideal birth are things which evolve magically out of the joy of being pregnant. Sadly, this is not the case. A happy, healthy pregnancy can be spoiled by unexpected and often unnecessary interventions during labour. An uninvolved, uninformed practitioner can turn otherwise straightforward ante-natal visits into a nightmare. The health of otherwise perfectly healthy babies can be compromised by the rushed or ill-considered medical diagnosis and treatment of their mothers.

Although the concepts of consumer choice and informed consent are much vaunted in the media, few women realize that they have any say at all about what happens to them ante-natally, during labour and afterwards. There is a great deal of research to show that a huge gap exists between the information which women want about pregnancy and childbirth, and the information which they get. Clearly, a woman who is having a baby is doing one of the most adult jobs of her life. She deserves access to accurate information – even if it challenges some of her own preconceived ideas – which might enable her to decide for herself about such basic issues as ante-natal testing, pain relief, where to give birth, who should be with her at the birth and where to go outside the hospital system for support.

The maternity services in Britain are slowly changing. There is a great deal of effort being made in the direction of de-medicalizing childbirth and forming a more mother-centred approach to maternity care. Unfortunately mothers are often the last to know about any changes made on their behalf, and the least well-informed about how they can shape their own individual birth experience. This book was written to fill the information gap.

The last two hundred years or so have seen women becoming less and less confident in their roles as birth-givers, and conversely more and more disconnected from the potential of pregnancy and birth.[1] We can't change history. But we can change what happens to us in the here and now. Anecdotal evidence suggests that women who are able to take responsibility for their pregnancy and birth are empowered far beyond these events. They are likely to be more confident parents. They are less predisposed to depression postnatally and able to tackle difficult issues – money, relationships, career and clashes with authority ranging from dealing with the benefits office to climbing the professional ladder – in a much more positive and self-assured manner.

Some of the information here might seem a little startling. Yet how differently might women view their maternity care if, for instance, they were aware that out of 100 common procedures carried out by obstetricians and midwives, around 20 are actually

Introduction

harmful?[2] Given evidence of this nature it would be easy to look upon some of the information here as confrontational or 'anti-doctor', or promoting some feminist tract. This would be missing the point. A woman doesn't need to be a 'feminist' to have a desire to inform herself and have some say in the type of care she receives. Nor does she have to be 'anti-doctor' to question or criticize those practices which may harm herself or her baby.

This is not just my personal view. The World Health Organization has made its position clear – 'Birth Is Not An Illness'. My late father might have put it more plainly – 'If it ain't broke, don't fix it!' Whatever clever way we choose to phrase it, the message is still the same: Birth is not a medical emergency. Pregnant women are not ill, though they are often treated as if they are. For instance, in her book *Women's Bodies, Women's Wisdom*, Dr Christiane Northrup recalls one night on the obstetrics ward when a pregnant woman was rushed unquestioningly from the casualty department up to the delivery suite. There, doctors discovered to their chagrin that the woman, who was in mid-pregnancy, had been seeking medical attention for a broken leg![3]

To help facilitate the idea of 'choice', pregnant women are often encouraged to think of themselves as consumers of maternity care. I agree with this philosophy, but recognize its many limitations. If you buy a car or a cooker and you are unhappy with it you can always take it back. If you have an upsetting birth experience, if you or your baby suffer or are damaged as a result of routine care, however well intentioned, you cannot make an exchange. You can't ask for your old body back or for a new baby. The truth is, you are only going to have this baby once, which is why it is important to choose the best possible care.

Maternity care issues highlight problems which are being faced throughout the medical world. These include the need to take doctors down from their pedestal, to begin to take responsibility for our own health, to de-escalate the technological and pharmacological war waged against our bodies, to inform patients of their rights and choices and to prevent, rather than continuously repair, damaged bodies.

Paradoxically, maternity care is also very different from other forms of care. A victim of a road accident may feel grateful for the efficient emergency care which a hospital can offer. He may be thankful for the range of drugs available, oblivious to the atmosphere of the room, indifferent about whether or not he likes the doctors or nurses attending him, and grateful for a bed in which to recover.

A pregnant woman, however, is alert, intelligent, and able to comprehend what is happening to her and around her. She may have strong feelings about the birth of her baby and about any drugs which may or may not be administered to her. She may, along with her partner, have wishes about the place of birth, her birth attendants and the environment her child is born in. She sees birth not as a medical event but as an individual and emotional experience as well as a social one.

This is primarily a book for and about mothers. It is meant to be read by women, their partners and their families. Its aim is to explain women's rights and choices in pregnancy and childbirth, but also to examine some of the things which influence the way women choose, as well as the possible consequences of those choices. I believe that most women instinctively know what is right for them and that the process of instinctual choice should be encouraged and supported. Nevertheless this is a book full of medical and practical information and quotes from a wide range of 'experts' (albeit 'mother-friendly' ones!). It is widely referenced and the information in it is based on widely accepted evidence. Use the information here to argue with your practitioner, if you feel you need to. But, frankly, if you have to quote chapter and verse to a doctor or midwife and argue every nuance of your care with them, you probably have the wrong doctor or midwife. Do yourself a favour and choose to move on.

In the end this book is best used as a resource, a place to turn to, a guide to getting the best out of what is on offer in the maternity services today. It does not promote the idea of orgasmic birth. I'm not even sure if this is possible, though some births – invariably those which have the least medical interference –

can be gentle and calm and loving. What this book looks towards are decent, humane births, births which leave women at least as healthy as they were before, and where women have a measure of control, some privacy and some dignity, are treated as individuals, and where their babies are treated like the precious beings they are. These things are really every woman's birthright.

Author's Note

Throughout this book I have referred to doctors as 'he' and midwives as 'she'. I am of course aware that there are female doctors and, less commonly, male midwives. My choice is, I believe, in keeping with the spirit and evidence-based nature of this book. In my mind there is no confusion between individual male doctors, some of whom are excellent, and the wider and more damaging 'masculine' ethos of obstetrics. I hope readers will recognize this. In addition, Health Service figures[4] show that out of more than 28,000 GPs in the UK, 40 per cent are female. This is substantial, but male GPs are still in the majority. Less encouraging is the fact that only 19 per cent of consultants are female.

Finally, I have a son, so my natural inclination would be to refer to all babies as 'he', even though the fashionable alternative is to call them 'she' or to alternate 'he' and 'she' between sentences, paragraphs, sub-sections or chapters. I have always thought this was a bit silly and very much beside the point, so have chosen to use the more neutral 'it' when referring to babies. My apologies to politically-correct fetuses everywhere!

1
Looking Ahead – Birth Options

Few women realize that the choice of where to give birth can affect their whole birth experience. It is unfortunate that women are often asked to make pronouncements about where they will give birth as soon as their pregnancy is confirmed, and usually before they have had a chance to fully consider all their options. Remember, this is one of the first, and biggest, decisions you may make and there is no need to hurry the process along. In fact, you and your baby may reap tangible benefits from taking the time to look ahead not only to your possible choices but to the consequences of these choices.

When considering where to give birth there is a tendency to draw battle lines – home birth versus hospital birth, natural birth versus medical birth. A vast amount of media attention has been focused on these issues and on the disagreements between mothers who would only have one and those who would only have the other. Not only is this very divisive, but it renders us blind to the range of options in between.

In reality there are many different possibilities open for a woman considering where and how to give birth. She may give birth in hospital with a short or long stay afterwards, with a familiar midwife at home, or on a Domino scheme. She may opt for an isolated or integrated GP unit or may prefer to labour and/or give birth in water at home or in hospital. She may opt out of the NHS altogether and employ an independent midwife or have private hospital care.

It's unfortunate that not all regions of Britain offer the same comprehensive range of choices. In Scotland, for instance, there are no practising independent midwives left. The combination of being unable to afford to insure themselves and the fact that Trusts there have refused independent midwives access to their facilities has effectively killed the profession. In Northern Ireland the few remaining GP units are being systematically shut down. Author Deborah Jackson, who has birthed her babies in Cardiff, Manchester and Bath, has noted the differences in care between each of these cities and mused, 'Some parents move house in order to send their children to a chosen school. I wonder how many consider the importance of locality on the kind of maternity care they will receive?'[1] Wherever you live, it behoves you to find out what is available in your area as early as possible. You can consult your GP or, if he is not helpful, your local Community Health Council for information about what facilities are available.

In the midst of these practicalities it is also important to have a wider perspective on birth which includes events leading up to and even beyond birth. So much of what women learn during pregnancy is focused on labour and birth that anybody could be forgiven for thinking that this is the main event before which and after which nothing matters. In reality birth, although a major event in its own right, is also just another stage in the continuum. Everything that happens before – including your own birth, your sexuality, conception and pregnancy – affects the choices you make and the way your baby's birth will be. The way the birth is will influence everything – your attitudes to mothering, sexuality, self-esteem and identity – which happens afterwards. For some women pregnancy and giving birth are opportunities to affirm strongly held beliefs. For others they offer a chance to break old patterns. Bringing this kind of consciousness to pregnancy and birth can make negotiating the many choices available somewhat easier.

Hospital Care

The vast majority of women are directed into the hospital system, whether they need to be or not and regardless of any preferences which they might have. Within the NHS there are two main types of hospitals: *consultant units* and *teaching hospitals*. It is usually assumed that a woman who books into a teaching hospital will, by virtue of the hospital's mandate for teaching students about the most recent developments in obstetrics, receive the most up-to date care available. But actually there is very little difference between the two types of units. In both places policy and practice will reflect the ethos of the senior consultant.

Whether you book into a consultant unit or teaching hospital, the routine will be much the same. These units have the highest rates of intervention during labour and statistically the poorest outcomes for mothers and babies. This has led one observer, who has carefully calculated the differences between birth in hospital and at home, to state that as many as 2400 babies die each year as a result of iatrogenic (the result of medical intervention) causes.[2]

Early on you will no doubt be told that the hospital's policy on interventions is not to use them routinely, but only when indicated. This may sound reassuring, but be aware that the phrase 'only when indicated' is open to a wide range of interpretations. It covers everything from deviation from the so-called 'normal' curve of labour (i.e. 'normal' duration of the first and second stages of labour and 'normal' strength and consistency of contractions) to 'normal' heart rhythms for the baby, 'requests' from the mothers for doctors to intervene, and whether or not the doctor or midwife is delivering someone else down the hall and needs to get on.

Even more interesting is that apparently the phrase 'only when indicated' can be influenced by something seemingly so trivial as the day of the week. It has been known for years that fewer babies are born on Sundays and public holidays than at any other time of the year, and that conversely births reach a peak in the weeks before longer holiday periods such as Christmas and Easter. The number of inductions of labour and caesarean operations is consistently higher on these days. In view of this the authors of one report conclude that this is not mere chance and that, '...it seems more likely (particularly in view of the disruption of the pattern seen at bank holidays) that the variation is a reflection of obstetric practice.'[3]

The only way to be sure if a hospital's stated policy is reflected in day-to-day practice is to get hold of their statistics for the last two years. You can do this by speaking to or applying in writing to the Supervisor of Midwifery. If the hospital is reluctant to give you this information, there are other avenues which you can try. Your local Community Health Council (CHC), if it's any good at all, should keep statistics on all the local hospitals. The CHC has a statutory right and a duty to obtain local hospital statistics in order to carry out its function as a watchdog for local health services.

If, however, you are stuck with a disinterested CHC or one which is taking too long to respond, you could also try your local branch of the National Childbirth Trust (NCT). Some groups keep a record of hospital statistics and even produce information booklets for mothers. If the figure for any procedure (monitoring, inductions, forceps, episiotomies, caesareans, etc.) is higher than 10 to 12 per cent, then you know that your local unit is intervening more often than is necessary. You do not have to make any decision about which hospital you would prefer (even though you may feel pressurized to do so) until you feel ready to.

Some consultant units tend to practise what is known as 'just in case' labour routines. These comprise of:

> Just in case your labour doesn't progress you will be induced. Just in case your baby has problems you will have

electronic fetal monitoring. Just in case the pain is too much you will have drugs. Just in case the baby is distressed you will have an episiotomy. Such attitudes create anxieties in the labour wards and result in an over-use of obstetric technology, much of which was developed to help mothers and babies with real problems but is often used routinely on mothers who do not have any – until they suffer unnecessary interventions.[4]

The just-in-case routines in consultant units place healthy mothers at an immediate disadvantage. This is because they get lumped in with all the high-risk mothers and there is a natural tendency for procedures which are only appropriate in obstetric emergencies to spill over into being used for normal women with normal babies.

If you do not find what you want in your area and there is another hospital within a reasonable distance from your home which you would prefer, you can always negotiate a place there. If the hospital of your choice is in another health district you can insist on an extra-contractual referral – a system by which the Purchasing Authority in your area pays for you to have care provided by another Trust. You do not have to go through your GP to do this, you can approach the hospital of your choice directly. However, a referral from your doctor may carry more weight with some more conservative units.

Take the hospital tour, by all means – you don't have to be pregnant to do this. But don't be fooled by attractive décor. Many hospitals are calling in interior decorators to make their birthing rooms look more 'homelike', resulting in a profusion of rooms which are often described as being like country hotels, 'with pine furniture, carpets and Laura Ashley fabrics'.[5] What those women whose homes do not resemble a country hotel are supposed to make of this is not clear.

The attempt to make hospitals more like hotels, in response to an increased demand for home births, misses the point entirely. Pretty wallpaper and nice curtains do not guarantee a normal birth, although they can exert a powerful effect on mothers, sometimes making them feel happier about the interventions they do receive. After all, a mother might reason, if the hospital has gone to so much trouble to provide an apparently low-tech atmosphere (the machines are there but usually kept out of sight in nice cabinets), then they must be taking an equal amount of trouble to provide a low-tech birth. If you walk into a birthing room and the bed is the most prominent piece of furniture (it's usually smack dab in the middle of the room), it is a pretty good indication that the pleasant surroundings are nothing more than a thin veneer to cover up fairly entrenched ideas about how and where women should give birth.

Talking to people can be helpful, but it can also be deceiving. We naturally want to trust our care-givers – so much so that we often miss what is really being said. The only way you will know for sure what your chosen hospital does and doesn't do is to take a look at its statistics. It can be a tedious job, but a rewarding one for any woman interested in getting the best possible care. The idea of shopping around for maternity care may seem a bit odd. But it's important to remember that you are a consumer of care, a hospital 'customer'. Hospitals want your business – they get paid somewhere in the region of £1800 for every baby they deliver. Bringing this kind of consumer consciousness to your choice of maternity care can help you to identify and prioritize your needs, making it easier to choose the care that is right for you and your baby.

GP or Midwife Units

GP Units (also known as Midwife Units or 'Home-from-Home' Units) are probably the closest thing we have within the NHS system to the birthing centres which are so popular in the US and Australia. They are usually small, they have a consistent record of fewer interventions in labour, and they are staffed and run by midwives who work closely with GPs.

Some GP units are free-standing centres, others are attached to larger consultant units. In other cases, what some doctors refer to as a GP unit is really just a certain number of beds, within a large consultant unit, allocated for the patients of local GPs (this is not a true GP unit).

In a GP unit women usually labour and give birth in the same room. It should be possible to bring personal items such as music, a bean bag, pictures or a favourite blanket along to make the rooms, which are often quite barren, more pleasant.

The UK government has stated that it is committed to returning maternity care to the community. But in practice many GP units are closing down, giving way to larger, more centralized hospital units which, it is argued, make better financial sense. Also, the differences in care between GP and consultant units appear to be narrowing, with many GP units adopting the active management protocols of larger consultant units.[6]

Still, if you have a GP unit in your area and wish to have a birth with as few interventions as possible (but are wary of having a home birth), they are worth investigating. Bear in mind, though, that standards of care in these units are by no means uniform.

There has been a great deal of research which shows that, for low-risk women, giving birth in a GP unit is as safe, and in some circumstances safer, than giving birth in a consultant unit.[7] Certainly over the years these units have proven their commitment to low-intervention care. Women in GP units are less likely to have inductions, augmentations, forceps deliveries, epidurals, pethidine and electronic fetal monitoring (EFM). One well-known study revealed that, for women having their first baby in a GP unit, EFM is used in 18 per cent of cases, and for women having their second or more baby it is used in only 3 per cent of cases. This compares with rates of 35 per cent and 19 per cent respectively in a consultant unit. Rates for the whole range of other interventions were shown to be double or more in consultant units. Babies fare better too in a GP unit. Fetal distress is twice as likely to be diagnosed in a consultant unit, and APGAR scores (the first physical assessment of the baby at one minute old) are better in GP units, with only 2 per cent of babies having a score of less than 6, as opposed to 18 per cent of babies born in consultant units.[8]

Don't, however, assume the safety and commitment to low-tech care of your local unit – you should always enquire about its rates for inductions, forceps, EFM, etc. before deciding.

Units which are free-standing and located away from larger hospitals have a better record for intervention-free birth than those which are located within a consultant unit. The idea behind those GP units attached to a consultant unit is that, if she needs additional help during labour, a woman can be transferred early to a place where there is a larger range of more sophisticated equipment. In these units the transfer rates are high and usually done on a 'just in case' basis. For a mother, being transferred from one unit to another in labour can be very confusing, disruptive and devastating to her confidence. Also, the babies of women who are transferred in labour have a higher rate of perinatal mortality (death). This may not be due to the lack of safety within a GP unit – the place of booking – but more to the higher rates of 'emergency' intervention on the newly transferred mother.[9]

What's more, it is unlikely that the people who have been caring for you in the GP unit will be able to go with you to the consultant unit. This means that you will have to deal with a whole new set of people at a time when you are at your most vulnerable. If you are considering booking into a GP unit, one of the most important questions you can ask is what percentage of women are transferred to hospital, and for what reason(s).

When a hospital makes beds available to GPs or midwives this usually means you will labour with your chosen GP or midwife, as long as labour progresses normally. Any deviation from what hospital policy defines as 'normal', however, generally means you will be transferred to a consultant's care.

Private Hospitals
The choice of a private hospital often has more to do with social status and aesthetic values than the quality of care on offer. The NHS provides a comprehensive service for all women, and the routine does not vary at all between private and NHS hospitals.

The majority of women booking private care are wealthier and in better health than most mothers in the UK. These facts alone would lead most observers to postulate that women choosing private care would be ideal candidates for a more natural birth with fewer interventions. But this is not the case. According to Beverley Lawrence Beech of the Association for Improvements in the Maternity Services (AIMS), many private hospitals would simply not be allowed to function within the NHS because their intervention rates and outcomes are so unsatisfactory. She maintains that:

> Choosing private maternity care does not necessarily ensure that you have an obstetrician attending your delivery nor does it mean that you will have a safer birth. On the contrary, private maternity units have the highest infant mortality rates, the highest morbidity rates and higher levels of litigation than any other area of maternity care. Private maternity units do, however, provide excellent hotel facilities. You will have your own private room, good food, and often a bottle of champagne provided following the birth.[10]

There are several other drawbacks to private care. It is impossible to say with any accuracy how 'safe' birth in a private hospital is – they are not under any obligation to produce statistics in the way that NHS hospitals are, and many simply do not. Also, not all of your care is paid for by private medical insurance. Only the non-routine and emergency interventions are covered, and this is bound to influence the way in which the hospital operates. The formula is simple: the more interventions which are used, the more money the hospital is paid. So there is a real tendency to give a woman everything going, whether she needs it or not, all in the name of the 'best possible care'.

In addition, the consultants in private hospitals are not as freely available as one might imagine. Obstetricians who work within the NHS and in private practice are obliged to devote the majority of their time to the NHS. So you may find that you are not attended by the consultant you are booked under any more often than you are in an NHS hospital. Private hospitals have high induction rates: You may find that the consultant tries to book you for an induction on a specific date – not because it is best for your baby, but because it is more convenient for his tight schedule.

Birthing Centres

There are very few independent birthing centres in the UK, unlike in the US and Australia. The ones which do exist tend to be run by the NHS or independent midwives. At a birthing centre you will have many of the facilities of a smaller GP unit and probably fewer interventions. Rooms will be pleasant and comfortable and there are usually extras like water pools to labour or give birth in. It is too early to evaluate the impact which centres like this will have on the general standard of care. But anything which gives women more choice can't be bad. If you plan to have your baby at a birthing centre, all your ante-natal care will be either at home or at the centre. Some even run their own antenatal classes. The cost may be prohibitive to some parents, but others may be in a position to consider it a sound investment physically, emotionally and financially. The Independent Midwives Association (IMA) can advise you about what is available in your area. Some CHCs and GPs may also have this information (*see also Appendix C*).

When Can You Leave?

Women who wish to give birth in hospital frequently ask 'When can I leave?' Those who wish to spend as little time as possible in the hospital environment are often given the option of a Domino scheme or a 6- or 48-hour discharge (*see below*). These schemes, though valuable, are also misleading in that their names imply that it is up to the doctor or midwife to say when you can go home. And as more and more hospitals are now operating early discharge systems, these types of schemes are fast becoming obsolete.

The truth is that you can discharge yourself and your baby from hospital at any time. You do not need permission from the doctor or midwife. Some hospitals refuse to discharge women because there is not an ambulance to take them home. You do not have to wait for an ambulance to take you home, however. You can go in your own car (although you will not be able to drive yourself after a caesarean operation), in a taxi, or by whatever method you choose. You do not need anyone to escort you, though in practice most women want (and it is probably wise) to have someone there.

If you wish to stay longer in hospital, your rights are less clear. Some units will not keep you longer than overnight unless there are complications. You do have some leverage, however. Find out (preferably before you give birth) what the 'common stay' (the average number of days a mother remains in hospital) is at your unit. You are then in a better position to negotiate to stay that long – but no longer. If you have compelling personal reasons for wanting to stay longer (for example your living conditions are stressful or you have no help arranged for yourself and the baby), you may also be able to arrange to stay longer. If your baby is ill and needs special care, you also have good reason to stay put, to breastfeed and help look after him (if your other family commitments will allow). Amazingly, in some units pressure will be brought on you to go, but some women have found simple stubborn refusal works wonders to bend the rules.

Domino Schemes
Domino stands for **Domicilary In** and **Out**, and is a very specific form of care. On a Domino scheme you are cared for by your local midwife in and out of hospital. She provides your antenatal care, sometimes independently, sometimes in tandem with your GP. You spend the early part of your labour at home with the midwife making periodic checks on you. Together, you and the midwife can determine when it is time to transfer to hospital for delivery. Your midwife cannot take you to hospital in her own car, so you will need to make other arrangements. You can

be driven by your husband or birth partner or, if you do not have access to transport, you can call an ambulance. Once you have given birth, you are free, usually after a couple of hours, to go home. Your midwife will continue to look after you for the statutory 10 days postnatally.

With the Domino scheme you will have the care of a midwife you know. By spending the early part of your labour at home you have a better chance of avoiding the number of interventions which women who go into hospital too early (an easy miscalculation to make, particularly the first time around) are subject to. There is generally no need for a woman in early labour to be in hospital anyway. She will be more comfortable and probably make better progress in her own home moving, eating, drinking and resting as she pleases and surrounded by familiar people and things.

Some hospitals do not operate their Domino schemes to the letter. For instance, they may ask a woman to come into hospital immediately she goes into labour. Once in hospital it may be the woman's own midwife who looks after her, or it may be hospital staff – the hospital decides. Having given birth, she is then discharged 6 hours or so later. This is not Domino care.

The Domino scheme, which has been around since the 1970s, is always promoted by doctors as being the ideal compromise between home and hospital delivery. But there has been surprisingly little evaluation of the scheme's effectiveness or of women's attitudes to it.

To be honest you do not have to book an 'official' Domino scheme to have this kind of delivery. This is because you are not obliged to tell the hospital or your midwife the moment you go into labour, even if you are instructed to. If you wish you can wait until your labour is established to summon the midwife or go to the hospital under your own steam or by ambulance. Having given birth, you have the right to discharge yourself and your baby at any time.

6- or 48-hour Discharge

There is no statutory time for which a mother must remain in hospital after the birth of her baby. Nevertheless, some hospitals operate schemes which offer mothers 'early' discharge, usually either within 6 or 48 hours of giving birth. If you choose to give birth in hospital and want your stay to be as short as possible, you can ask for one of these bookings. They should be made available to anyone – even mothers who have had caesareans. The 6- or 48-hour time limits are entirely arbitrary and exist mainly to fit in with hospital routines, midwifery staffing levels, the reality of too few beds and cost-cutting exercises. You can ask to be discharged, or discharge yourself, at any interval in between. Provided you and your baby are fit and well and you feel confident that you can manage at home, there should be no pressure put upon you to stay.

What Can You Eat?

Many hospitals refuse to let women eat and drink in labour – preferring instead to keep them hydrated and their blood sugar levels up by using an intravenous drip of water and glucose (also known as dextrose). One reason for this is that vomiting and diarrhoea are a natural part of labour for some women and can occur early on as well as in the transition phase, and hospitals like to keep the 'birth environment' as clean as possible 'for the baby's sake' and so that the mother can avoid 'embarrassment'. Another reason for withholding food is just in case a general anaesthetic needs to be performed. Under these circumstances there is a risk a mother might inhale her own vomit, which can result in respiratory problems or, very rarely, death. When this happens it is always because the anaesthetist has not followed the correct procedure (see Chapter 5) – no woman who has been properly anaesthetized has ever inhaled her own vomit. In any case, the necessity for a general anaesthetic is so rare that it hardly justifies the widespread policy of starvation during labour.

There has yet to be any scientific assessment of women's nutritional needs during labour. But based on what is known, there is *no evidence* that denying food and drink to a woman doing the hardest, most physical job of her life serves any useful purpose. The problem is that, denied proper fuel, your muscles cannot work efficiently. The uterus is a muscle, and glucose provides the energy which it, and all your other muscles, need while working so hard in labour. If the body is short of glucose because of fasting it will burn other fuel such as fat. If this goes on for some time you become ketotic. Ketones – the acidic products of fat metabolism – appear in the blood and are a sign of exhaustion. A mother may, of course, choose to avoid the possibility of vomiting and/or diarrhoea by not eating, but this choice needs to be weighed carefully against the possibility of denying her body the essential fuel needed to cope with labour.

There is also some evidence to show that a drip may be harmful to your baby. The dextrose solutions used in labour can cross the placenta, resulting in abnormally high blood sugar levels in newborn babies. Because these blood sugar levels cannot be maintained after birth the baby then experiences the shock of hypoglycaemia (a drop in blood sugar to abnormally low levels).

Although most women do not want to eat, particularly in the later stages of labour, the choice of eating and drinking freely, particularly early on, should be entirely theirs. A very few enlightened hospitals now have a menu of suitable food and drink for labouring women. However, if you are in one of the many units in Britain that does not look favourably upon food during labour, you should know that you have the right to insist on eating and can, if you wish, bring your own food (though in some cases pressure will be put upon you not to). A drip, with all its discomfort and potential side-effects, can be avoided if you are able to maintain your fluid balance and blood sugar levels with fruit juices, herbal tea with honey, and light snacks such as clear broth, crisp buttered toast, lightly boiled eggs and cooked fruits.

Home Birth

Every woman has the legal right to give birth at home, regardless of whether she is expecting her first or subsequent child and regardless of what her perceived 'risk' factor is. If you opt for a home birth your local health authority has a legal obligation to make sure that you are attended by a qualified practitioner, usually a midwife. No practitioner can force you to sign a waiver relinquishing him of all responsibility for any 'bad' outcome. In any case these waivers are not legally binding, and it is interesting to note that no doctor has ever signed a piece of paper guaranteeing the safety of a hospital birth. The decision to give birth at home rests solely with the individual mother and is not dependent on anybody else – GP, midwife or consultant – giving his permission. This fact is still not widely appreciated or understood. Many women still talk about 'not being allowed' a home birth, or complain 'they do not do home births in my area.'

For a woman, choosing a home birth may simply be a matter of acknowledging her needs for privacy, security, comfort, safety, control, freedom and respect for the emotional and spiritual aspects of birth. She may have had a previous bad experience in hospital and wish to avoid another. She may wish to avoid unnecessary interventions, or have a desire to put birth back into the context of a family event, to improve the quality of her early contact with her baby and ensure the establishment of breastfeeding. For some, more practical reasons may prevail, such as being a long way from the nearest hospital.

For some doctors and midwives, being confronted with a woman wanting a home birth is a complex, even frightening thing which represents a real challenge to their authority. For instance, even though the majority of GPs do not attend births and have never seen a normal birth, for a woman actively to choose to exclude her GP by booking a home birth directly with a midwife is felt as a slap in the face. Equally, many midwives are not confident of their skills and as a result are uncomfortable with the idea of home birth. When they do reluctantly attend home births, they feel as if they are on alien territory, as if they are not in control, that they are outnumbered and don't know where anything is – in fact, ironically, all the things which a woman may feel when she is in hospital.

Some professionals belittle home birth as merely a middle-class fad, but the experience of practitioners, both GPs and midwives, with working-class clientele suggests otherwise. A group of GPs who have been attending home births in the UK for 12 years comment that 'Birth at home may seem to be an interest of the eccentric middle class, but our experience is that an appreciable number of working class women will opt for home birth *if the service is available* [my emphasis].'[11] Equally, a pioneering group of midwives in South East London with a 75 per cent home birth rate (as opposed to 1.8 per cent nationally) note that 'A third of our clients are on benefits and many more are grappling with heavy socio-economic pressures.'[12] This group, which has contracted into the NHS, reserves most of its services for women who are often denied choice within the health service, including those from ethnic minorities, those considered to be high-risk and those with mental or physical disabilities. Yet in addition to a high home birth rate, these mothers go on to achieve a rate of spontaneous vaginal delivery in 87 per cent of cases, and a caesarean rate which is less than half the national average. In addition, 74 per cent need no pain relief during labour, and the rates for breastfeeding 28 days after birth stand at 96 per cent, as compared with the national average of 25 per cent.

When you opt for a home birth you are taking control. You are accepting responsibility for the outcome, good or bad (although your carer is always liable for negligence). There are very few societal rewards at the moment for women who choose to give birth at home. But the personal rewards, as borne out by the statistics – safety, control, a sense of achievement, healthier mother and baby – more than make up for this.

Looking Ahead – Birth Options

Booking a Home Birth

Unfortunately, booking a home birth is likely to be an obstacle course unless you have enough financial resources to book with an independent midwife. Private midwives are the most experienced practitioners when it comes to home births. You can be reassured by the fact that they often don't do anything else. Booking a home birth via the NHS should be just as straightforward – but it rarely is.

Because the GP is usually the first place a woman goes when she is pregnant, many women make the natural mistake of going along to the surgery and asking about home birth. In the majority of cases they will be told they can't have one. The GP's surgery is the first hurdle at which the majority of mothers fall. The government report *Changing Childbirth* makes it clear to practitioners that 'GPs who feel unable to offer care or support to a woman who wishes to have a home birth should refer the woman directly to a midwife.'[13] In practice, though, many don't – perhaps because GPs do not get paid if they refer a woman on to midwifery care.

There is no reason – medical, legal or ethical – to involve your GP at all if you want a home birth. So few GPs are experienced in home deliveries (in fact, in deliveries of any kind) that any confrontation with your GP may end up just wasting your time and his.

If you want a home birth your first point of contact should be the Supervisor of Midwives at your local hospital. You can do this by phone or letter, though a letter has the advantage of recording your request officially. If you write a letter, keep a copy.

Your booking visit will be at home – you may be visited by the midwives who will attend you or by the Supervisor herself. Usually if the Supervisor comes it's to talk you out of your decision or to explain why you can't have a home birth. Don't be put off. The reluctance of healthcare personnel is not a legitimate reason for any woman to be refused a home birth if this is what she wants.

Having booked a home birth, your ante-natal care should be at a local clinic or, if you prefer, you can ask for it to take place in your home with a community midwife – some are happy to do this. Any attempt to get you to accept an appointment at the local hospital should be viewed with suspicion. This is invariably so that the consultant can try to convince you of the error of your ways. If there is no good reason to go to a hospital appointment, don't. You are not legally obliged to attend. Some women are asked to go to the hospital to discuss the results of early screening tests. Once in hospital they are told that everything looks fine but ... 'I see you are wanting a home birth – do you think this is wise?' The consultant does not need to approve a home confinement, nor can he refuse to provide one.

Many doctors and midwives will tell you that birth is only safe in retrospect. This is not true. Too many professionals have never seen a birth without interventions and without the backstop of the institution behind them, and this frightens them. If your doctor or midwife is not supportive of your desire to have a home birth – move on. Don't waste precious time and energy trying to convince him or her that you are right. Life is too short – and pregnancy is even shorter.

You do not have to enter into a dialogue. You do not have to justify your choice or produce reasons or evidence to substantiate it. In fact you do not have to say anything more substantial than 'because I want to' in response to any questions about why you want to give birth at home. You may even be asked to sign a disclaimer – this is a tremendously effective form of emotional blackmail but has no standing in law and you are not obliged to sign it. If you do decide to sign anyway you can always do so with the proviso that you can insert the words 'I am signing this because of the emotional pressure to do so applied by ... [insert the name and title of your doctor and/or midwife]' at the bottom. Under these circumstances it's important to name names.

Even though the initial visit is in your home, and therefore on your territory, you may wish to have your partner or a friend with you. A midwife once confided in me that she usually

Looking Ahead – Birth Options

brought another midwife along with her when she visited mothers, so that if there was ever any dispute about what had been said, she would have someone to back her up. She then added that 'pregnant women don't always listen very well!' If the 'buddy system' can work for the health service, it can work for you too!

You may be worried that you can't find GP cover for a home birth. Relax – it is not your job to find a doctor who will agree to cover a home birth. Having booked directly with the midwife, should she feel that you will need GP cover it is up to her to arrange it.

Home Birth Safety
In spite of evidence to the contrary, there is still a lot of scepticism about the safety of home birth. GPs can get hot under the collar when faced with a woman who wants a home birth. Midwives, too, can become obstructive and officious. The kind of opposition you can expect includes comments like:

✷ What will happen if something goes wrong and your baby dies? How will you feel then?

✷ What will happen if you die? Who will look after your baby?

✷ You can't have a home birth with a first baby because you have an untried pelvis (one that hasn't had a baby pass through it yet).

✷ Have your baby at home if you want, but I can't possibly provide cover for you in an emergency.

✷ If you'd ever seen a post-partum haemorrhage you would never risk such a thing.

✷ What if we had to call the flying squad out while it was dealing with someone who was dying?

* Birth is so messy – you might ruin the carpet.

* We are very short staffed at the hospital, and if we cover you at home it will be at the expense of other mothers having their babies in hospital.

* Wouldn't you feel guilty if you took the flying squad away from the hospital where they are really needed?

* You know you can't have an epidural at home?

In addition, women are told that it is wrong for them to 'play God', that they can't predict what will happen, that their obstetric histories are poor, that their blood pressure is too high, that they are anaemic, that they have 'gestational diabetes', that it is only safe with your second baby, not the first (or third or fourth or more). Most of these arguments are simply nonsense.

Many women who are confronted with these kinds of excuses feel they have nowhere to turn. They wonder whether anyone would even believe them if they repeated some of the extraordinary things which medical practitioners have said to them. Getting in touch with organizations such as AIMS and the NCT (*see Appendix C*), who have heard it all before, can be a great source of support. They are always prepared to listen and believe women's stories about the difficulties of getting the kind of birth they want.

Statistics suggest that planned home births are the safest births of all. They produce the smallest number of low birthweight babies: only 2.5 per cent of home birth babies weigh less than 2,500 g (5^1/$_2$ lb), as opposed to 18 per cent of those born in hospital.[14] They have the lowest overall rate of perinatal mortality (stillbirth and death up to six days after birth). The national rate is 8.9 per 1,000 but the rate for home births is 4.3 per 1,000. Moreover, half of those babies who die at home would have died wherever they were born due to severe congenital abnormalities or very low birthweight. This has prompted the opinion that 'If the objective is to reduce perinatal mortality as quickly as possible, all the evidence already accumulated indicates most cogently that the most immediate and effective method would be to reverse the policy which seeks to ensure that all births take place in obstetric hospitals.'[15]

One general practice which has been delivering babies at home for more than a decade reported that, out of 285 women booked for a home delivery, only one death occurred at 39 weeks 'without warning and before the onset of labour, after an uneventful pregnancy'. Only two babies born at home weighed less that 2,500 g (5^1/$_2$ lb).[16]

These kinds of results are not unique to the UK. In the US, The Farm (a self-sufficient community where babies are delivered by midwives, at home, in over 90 per cent of cases) now commands the highest safety record in the country. A report of The Farm's 1,888 births between 1970 and 1994 showed that in 24 years only 11 babies died from neonatal complications; of these, four had lethal congenital defects.[17]

Nobody who has read the available evidence on the safety of home birth in relation to birth elsewhere could rationally rule out home birth on the grounds of safety. It has been shown again and again that home birth is as safe, and for women in a 'low-risk' category, may even be safer, than hospital birth.

Why then are there so few home births? Certainly not because of lack of interest from mothers. A recent NCT survey concluded that 'the home birth rate is increasing where women are given a real choice.'[18] According to the most recent government report,[19] a MORI poll commissioned to find out women's attitudes to choice revealed that 22 per cent of those who expressed a preference wanted a home birth. This represents an overall figure of 16 per cent of all mothers. Yet less than 2 per cent actually achieve their goal. This is not because most transfer to hospital, give birth to dead babies or die in the effort. Even if we assume that 10 per cent of these mothers may transfer to hospital for delivery, this leaves us with a substantial proportion of women who want, but do not achieve, a home birth, probably due to misinformation or lack of support from their practitioners.

The intriguing question, then, may be for whom is home birth 'unsafe'? It is tempting to propose that the people who are the most 'at risk' during a home birth are our doctors and midwives. As Campbell and Macfarlane comment:

> The stated rationale of a policy that all women should give birth in hospital is that this affords the safest environment. Unlike home, hospitals for most women are alien environments over which they have almost no control. This is not true for obstetricians and hospital midwives. Thus it might be suggested that when obstetricians recommend that the wishes of women should be met, but only 'within the confines of safety', this means – at least in part – within the confines of an environment in which the obstetrician feels safe.'[20]

A mother who wants a home birth should also consider how 'safe' she will be in the hands of a practitioner who has no experience of home birth. If you are not confident about your midwife's skill, write to the Supervisor of Midwives immediately with your concerns, and insist that she replace your midwife with another who is both skilled and enthusiastic about home birth. She is legally obliged to do this, so don't take no for an answer.

Who Should Be There?

Birth is an intensely personal event. Who will be with you during labour is a question which cannot be answered simply. While birthing women remain relatively constant, trends are constantly changing around them. There was a time when the father's experience of birth was pacing up and down in the waiting room or, for some, at the pub. Children were dispatched to the nearest relative, friend or neighbour, and the mother was left alone to 'get on with it'. Today a great deal of social pressure is put on fathers to be there – a trend which does not suit all fathers or mothers.

Looking Ahead – Birth Options

Women should be encouraged to take this idea on board and to think carefully about who will (and will not) be with them during this time.

Other Adults
Women should be free to choose who and how many of their nearest and dearest should be with them at the birth. But this is not always the case. If you choose a hospital birth there may be restrictions on whom you can bring with you. Certainly you will not automatically be allowed to have your other children there. Some hospitals are still a bit Draconian about allowing anybody other than, or instead of, your husband or male partner to be with you. Many practitioners actively resent the presence of others, believing that they only get in the way. A news release from the Royal College of Midwives commented that birth is 'fast becoming a growing spectator sport' and that midwives often can't get near a labouring mother for hoards of people waving red scarves and yelling 'push, push ... you'll never push alone.'[21] An odd point of view, since it is usually the practitioners who outnumber family members. To a woman it's probably anonymous staff members, and not her family, who are the real outsiders.

In assessing the problems caused by too many visitors, one study concluded that in 70 per cent of cases the biggest problem which staff members face is abusiveness and uncooperativeness.[22] Though it might seem obvious to some, the author of the study was at a loss to explain the cause of this behaviour. Hospitals are strange places, where the expectation of disaster is just around the corner. In hospitals people naturally feel anxious and helpless, and this can eventually translate into bad temper, rudeness and occasionally violence.

A woman who wants a large number of her family members present should consider how well each of them might react to the tense atmosphere of the hospital and any resentment which they may encounter from staff members. The level of anxiety of those around her will have a profound effect on her labour.

Too often a woman has no say in who is present for all or part of her labour. Hospital personnel work in shifts. A woman coming in halfway through a shift may find that at some point in her labour the faces around her change. Strangers can come and go with amazing regularity. One study, aiming to assess the frequency and ways in which personnel enter the rooms on a labour ward, found that 41 per cent of the time staff either entered without knocking or knocked as they entered – a result made even more surprising by the fact that doctors and midwives at this particular hospital were told beforehand that their behaviour was going to be monitored. 'We tend to think of hospitals as organized places,' writes the author, 'but often what is needed in labour, a gown, a pillow, a special piece of equipment, a drink of water, is not in the room.'[23] Commenting on the report's findings, Caroline Flint, President of the Royal College of Midwives, recalled a time when she was on a labour ward from 8 a.m. to 2 p.m. and '35 different people entered the room including the electrician to mend the bell, and the domestic to stock the shelves.'[24]

Some experts, such as Michel Odent, believe that women should be given the freedom to be alone for long periods during labour. He cites the behaviour of other animals who instinctively seek the darkest, most secluded places to give birth.

In actual fact, while you are in labour there may be times when you want to have someone there and times when you wish to be alone. It can be very hard to achieve this delicate balance if you are giving birth in hospital. For a woman giving birth at home it's less of a problem. You can have as many or as few people around as you want. Chances are you will naturally have extended periods of solitude because your midwives will probably be operating a system of periodic checks, coming to your house every few hours or so during early labour to assess your progress. In addition, your birth partner(s) can comfortably busy themselves elsewhere when you need to be alone.

It is usually assumed that a woman's birth partner will be her husband. In the majority of cases this may be true. But not all husbands are enthusiastic about 'being there'. Equally, not all women are enthusiastic about having their husbands with them. You should be aware that in hospital you have no legal right to have *anybody* there with you. But today hospitals universally recognize the moral right of the father, or chosen birth partner, to attend the birth, though some are less enthusiastic about allowing female partners in.

The only laws which exist about who should be with you at the birth are written in a very negative sense. In other words, the law says that it is illegal for anyone except a qualified midwife or doctor to deliver a baby, except in an emergency. In fact, any doctor can legally deliver a baby, even if he has no experience of doing so. It is, however, illegal for any woman to have her baby delivered by an unqualified person, such as her mother or husband, no matter how experienced he or she may be. Oddly enough, it is not illegal for a woman to give birth on her own (though it is unwise). Some women, however, have turned to this option in desperation, because it has been the only way they could achieve the kind of birth they wanted. No woman should be forced into giving birth alone, even though some do so without undue harm to themselves or their babies.

There is no one correct answer to the question about which adult members of your family and/or which of your friends you should have with you. Every mother needs to be guided by her inclinations and flexible enough to recognize that these might change during the course of her pregnancy. Her family and friends, however much they may want to be there, should respect her decision to include some and exclude others, as well as her right to amend that decision at any time.

Other Children
For a woman at home who has other children there is always the nagging question of whether the children should be at the birth. Much will depend on the individual family and their attitudes to sex and reproduction. Not all childbirth educators believe that having siblings at the birth is a good idea. There is argument that it can negatively affect children, particularly those who are

young and/or emotionally immature. For some mothers, having a child there can mean she may feel inhibited and unable to surrender to the demands of labour while she is worrying about the child's welfare.

However, those who like the idea believe that to include other children in the birth contributes greatly to the 'atmosphere of normalcy and family closeness'.[25] While there is no simple answer to the question of children at the birth, parents should examine carefully their motives for wanting the child there and should never force a child who is hesitant or unready to attend on the basis that it might be good for them. There are, however, some basic guidelines to help make birth a positive experience for a child. Ideally, these should be met before parents take the decision to have their other child(ren) there:

* The parents must be prepared for the birth. They need to have an understanding of the physiology of birth as well as its emotional and sexual nature. They must be confident about their ability to respond appropriately to its demands, otherwise their lack of confidence can affect the child's perception of the event.

* Your practitioner must be amenable to the idea. Check on this well in advance. Take the child with you to ante-natal clinic so that he or she can get to know your practitioner as well.

* Both parents should want their child(ren) to be there and the child(ren) should also want to be there. If a child is reluctant or uneasy, this should be respected.

* Parents must be aware of the child's emotional and physical state. A child who is ill will probably not be able to meet the emotional and physical demands of being a part of labour and birth. A child who has had a recent traumatic or frightening experience, particularly in

relation to his or her body, doctors or hospitals, may be even more traumatized by witnessing birth.

* The child must be prepared for the way birth is. This entails lots of open family discussions about what to expect. In addition, the child must be comfortable with a wide range of emotions and with seeing mother naked.

* The child must have an adult companion whose job is solely to provide support, reassurance, comfort and explanations as necessary. This should be someone whom the child knows and trusts.

* Parents must be flexible enough to respond if the child changes his or her mind, becomes unwell, is asleep or if labour complications develop which may require transfer to hospital. Prior explanation to the child and lots of nurturing are essential under these circumstances.

Be realistic about your child. Don't expect a toddler to be immediately moved or transformed by labour and birth. Children don't suddenly become more adult, calmer and more in tune with the universal, spiritual or sexual nature of birth. Be prepared for your child to need someone to wipe a bottom or a nose, to be hungry or grumpy, to say 'no', argue and fuss, to need cuddling and want to show you something or know where his or her favourite *Postman Pat* video is.

In her book *The Fun Starts Here*, Paula Yates describes her experience this way:

> Fifi was present while her new sister was born. She was a very active participant, standing on a chair next to the bed, shouting 'Push, push, push' like a very small cox on the Oxford and Cambridge Boat Race. She mainly wanted me to hurry so that she could eat the mint which had fallen down the side of the bed. Peaches was born, looking perfect

and gorgeous, like a little peach. The doctor said it was a girl. Fifi fell off her chair, cheering and came over to my bed. 'Can I have my mint now?' she asked.[26]

Giving Birth in Different Positions

Freedom of movement is one of the most important things in labour. Trials show that women who are given the freedom to move around will adopt several different positions during the second stage of labour. More than 33 per cent of women will adopt three or more different positions during labour, while 45 per cent will try at least two. This makes a striking comparison to women who are instructed to lie down, where 55 per cent simply obey and remain down and only 5 per cent try three or more positions.[27] Much of the available research shows a dogmatic search for the single 'right' position in which to give birth, whether it be lying down, semi-recumbent, standing upright or squatting. In the end there may not be a 'right' position, because every woman's needs are different and every labour progresses differently. There are, however, some well-demonstrated benefits of maintaining an upright position in preference to a horizontal one.

A woman who has the freedom to move around during the early stages of labour and who can adopt several different positions during the second, pushing stage of labour is doing for herself what obstetric drugs claim to do for her. She is helping to strengthen her contractions and make them more efficient; she is reducing the degree of pain experienced in a supine position, caused by the weight of the baby pressing against the sacral nerves; and she is working *with* her body and gravity instead of against them.

Walking in Early Labour
Ambulation, or walking through labour, has no known side-effects and, based on available evidence, appears to be as effective as the drug syntocinon for augmenting labour.[28] When the

contractions in the first stage of labour become strong enough, many women find that walking, standing or leaning forward is an effective way of managing them. Walking and standing promote a shorter labour, better all-round circulation and, because of this, an ultimately less tiring and painful labour.[29]

Results of controlled trials show that women who walk, stand or sit upright during labour usually have shorter labours than women who lie flat.[30] This may be because gravity ensures that the weight of the baby presses firmly against the cervix. This pressure signals the body's release of oxytocin, which improves the regularity and consistency of contractions.[31]

If you have stairs in your home you might try climbing them (also an effective method for dealing with a slow or halted labour), or you may enjoy dancing with your partner, or maybe you will prefer to be on your own, rotating your hips or rocking back and forth as your contractions become increasingly stronger.

You may be jittery and full of anticipation during early labour. Use this energy to your advantage if you can. It can be difficult for women giving birth in hospital to have the freedom of movement which they might want. Everything about the hospital routine seems to conspire to keep a woman lying down from the minute she enters the hospital door. But there is no reason at all why you should not remain active, if this is what you want. If you are in hospital walk the corridors, go to the toilet frequently, move in any way you can. If you are at home, just get on with your normal activities. Do the dishes, cook a meal, take the dog for a walk or go to the corner shop for a magazine. Walking will help move your labour along and will also help establish labour in the context of a normal life event.

In Western society we have a long history of thinking that labouring women are weak and incapable. This view is reinforced by the images in movies and on TV of distraught women lying on their backs from the first signs of labour until the first cry of their newborn babies.

When I was in labour I can remember my midwife constantly encouraging me to keep moving. At first this seemed an impossible demand. It was a struggle to get up on my feet. Then by chance a dreadful movie came on the TV in which a woman was labouring on her back screaming, crying, hurling abuse at her husband and surrounded by bright lights and people in masks and gowns. That was all I needed to pull myself up. The struggle to get up on your feet is not just a struggle against gravity, pain or exhaustion. It's a struggle against decades of prejudice and popular culture. First-time mothers, who have little or no idea of how labour really is, may unconsciously emulate any over-dramatized, second-hand images they have seen in magazines or films. Women interested in having a degree of control over their own births need to be wary of the insidious way in which popular media images of labouring women can influence their beliefs about their ability to give birth unaided, and consequently about their behaviour in labour. You can and should insist on being mobile during labour – even if your carers have other ideas.

Lying Down and Semi-recumbent
In spite of evidence against it, lying down, known as the lithotomy or supine position, continues to be the standard policy in many maternity units. Many practitioners still insist that women under their care lie down and stay down. There is no evidence to suggest that this is best for either mother or baby. A woman lying down or even semi-recumbent (lying at a 45 degree angle) is decreasing the flow of blood to the placenta, a possible cause of fetal distress because the baby is receiving less blood and oxygen. She is also decreasing the amount of blood available to the uterus, and less blood means less powerful contractions. In addition, because the uterus tilts forward during contractions, a woman lying down is effectively asking her uterus to work twice as hard to achieve the same results.

In women the coccyx, or tailbone, is hinged to order to increase the dimensions of the pelvic outlet during labour and allow greater ease in the delivery of a baby. Lying down or sitting on your backside means the potential dimensions of the pelvic outlet are restricted, sometimes by as much as 10 to 30 per cent.

The semi-recumbent position which so many hospitals favour for labour represents a kind of medical compromise. Many practitioners refer to it as a semi-squat. In reality it is a semi-lie down. Whatever name it's given, the consequences for women are the same. They tend to have longer labours and more pain, resulting in a greater tendency for them to be offered, and to accept, drugs to speed up labour and/or relieve pain.

Women who lie on their sides seem to be the one exception to the 'never lie down' rule. Many find this a comfortable position to be in, particularly if they are very tired. Available evidence seems to suggest that there is no difference in the length of labour between women in this lateral position and those who are upright.

Standing, Squatting and Sitting
In contrast to those women who choose to give birth lying down, those who give birth in an upright position use less pain-relieving drugs, have fewer epidurals and fewer drugs to augment labour. Women in an upright position also report feeling more satisfaction with the process and a greater feeling of having been in control.[32]

In traditional societies women usually give birth squatting, or standing, either supported by their attendants or supporting themselves by means of a rope or bar. The dwindling numbers of women giving birth in an upright position has come about as a result of doctors wishing to observe and manage women's labour. Early delivery tables had wrist, shoulder and leg straps in order to make sure that labouring mothers were completely immobilized. In the US, stirrups and leg supports are still used.

In spite of the huge amount of anecdotal evidence which suggests that an upright position is more advantageous to women, there is very little scientific data to show the benefits of maintaining an upright position for birth. This is partially because the ethics of randomly allocating women to a group which must either lie down or stay upright are questionable and constitute a basic infringement of their personal liberties with regard to the freedom of movement.

Active Birth pioneer Janet Balaskas maintains that an upright position, particularly one in which the woman is squatting, can enlarge the pelvic opening by as much as 20 per cent.[33] Others put the figure as high as 30 per cent.[34] The squatting position is one of the earliest recorded positions and is depicted in birth scenes dating back to several millennia BC. Many 'civilized' women find this a difficult position to get into and to maintain. A less active lifestyle, high-heeled shoes and even unexpected things like using toilets instead of squatting to defecate means that our ankles have lost their strength and flexibility.

Any woman, particularly one who is pregnant, who tries to get into a squat for the first time may find that she simply topples over. Yoga during pregnancy can help to improve strength and flexibility and help the mother find her 'centre of gravity', but some may still find it difficult to get into the squatting position without help. Even women who are physically able to squat may find that it increases the strength of contractions to the point where they are unbearable, or that they are simply too tired near the end of the second stage to maintain the position for long.

Some women are able to maintain a squat or true semi-squat with help and support from their birth attendants. Others prefer to try and support themselves by using a birth stool. The definition of a birth stool can include anything from a child's stool to a specially designed apparatus which has a horse-shoe shape cut out of it to allow delivery. One big disadvantage of the birth stool is that the mother is sitting on her tailbone and restricting its movement. It may be that a birth stool is more useful early in labour as a way of strengthening contractions, but less so in the pushing stage when a mother will need those extra couple of centimetres that a supported squat gives to aid delivery.

In response to women's desire to remain upright in labour, hospitals often provide birth chairs and birth beds. Most recently birth wheels – which look like giant gyroscopes left over from the set of *Barbarella* – have been introduced into European hospitals. All of these represent a kind of compromise between women's need for greater freedom of movement and practitioners' need for control in a hospital environment. A birth chair is a kind of articulated bed with parts that move into different angles, and sometimes a squatting bar to help a woman balance herself. Unfortunately these chairs are usually quite high off the ground and can cause the mother to feel inhibited and off balance.

There are lots of different types of birthing chairs. Some are relatively benign, with a hole cut into the bottom so the baby can be delivered easily into the hands of an attendant. Others are more menacing, with shoulder, ankle and wrist straps to restrain a woman during painful obstetric interventions.

Birth chairs are designed so that the mother is well supported in a nearly upright position with her legs apart and knees bent. The drawback is that the mother must adopt whatever position the manufacturer feels is the optimum position for birth, and this may not coincide with her own inclinations. In theory the chairs are designed so that the mother can operate controls to change the position of the chair to suit her needs, but in practice her attendants are in control, so freedom of movement may be more restricted than if the mother were simply to arrange herself over a bean bag, or on a bed or a chair with or without the support of her companions.

Often birth chairs are covered in practical material, such as vinyl, and while this makes them easy to clean it can be terribly uncomfortable for a hot, sweaty, labouring mother whose skin may feel extra-sensitive to all but the gentlest touch and the softest materials.

The only randomized trial to assess the benefits of a birth chair as opposed to 'bed birth' has produced disappointing, if somewhat predictable, results. It failed to prove any benefit from delivery in a birth chair, despite the mothers being in an upright position. There was even a small increase in the rate of postpartum haemorrhage for women using the chair. There was little difference in the rates of damage to the perineum, because the rates for episiotomy in the bed birth group were offset by the rates of tears in the birth chair group. More women in the chair group, though, did ultimately emerge with an intact perineum, perhaps because they were more upright.[35]

Further studies have shown that for women using birth chairs over long periods of labour there is an increased risk of perineal oedema (swelling) and haemorrhoids.[36] Among both women allocated to the lying down group and those allocated to the birth chair group, there was a marked ambivalence in response to the questions of satisfaction, comfort and feelings of control. This is probably because the women had no choice in their overall mode of delivery. The use of the birth chair does not appear to shorten the length of either the first or second stage of labour.

Water Labour, Water Birth

The healing, soothing, pain-relieving properties of water have been known about for centuries. For a woman in labour, water – hot or cold, running or still, poured, sprayed or splashed – can be a blessing. Some don't even need to be in the water to benefit from it. They just like the sound of it during contractions and will run the taps or the shower or flush the toilet over and over again, or play pre-recorded sounds of the ocean or running streams just to hear the soothing sound of water!

There has been a great deal of controversy in the press recently about what is loosely known as 'water birth'. A few reports of babies being born dead or brain damaged have caused some mothers to shy away from asking for the use of the water pools which many hospitals now have. As usual, these reports have been blown out of all proportion – but they have given everybody cause to think again about what exactly we mean when we say water birth.

First of all, when speaking about water birth we need to be clear whether we are talking about labouring in water, or labouring and giving birth in water. We also need to know that, while

Looking Ahead – Birth Options

many hospitals have responded to women's desire to labour in water by installing birthing pools, or by allowing women, at their own expense, to bring rented pools into a specially dedicated room at the hospital, they have not, unfortunately, made the corresponding effort to ensure that their staff are adequately trained in how best to use them. Neither have they kept up an adequate number of labours and/or births in each pool to ensure that staff maintain their levels of expertise. In addition, they haven't proved very enthusiastic about the idea of women renting pools for use in home births.

When something simple like a birthing pool comes into the hospital system, it becomes subject to operational guidelines and the women who want to use it must meet certain criteria. While it is not unreasonable that certain precautions should be taken, and that staff should be trained in how to get the best out of the equipment, it is unfortunate that not all hospitals follow the same rules or apply those which do exist in the same way. With this in mind, it was only a matter of time before some tragedy befell a mother or baby while giving birth in water. The handful of adverse reports about water birth which appeared during 1993/94 are a testimony to this.

Labour and/or birth in water is not a form of 'treatment', and as such one would not expect it to go through the rigorous assessment which a new drug, piece of equipment, or invasive procedure should go through. Nevertheless, the idea of water labour and water birth have been so under-evaluated that what evidence does exist is based on anecdotal accounts and a handful of small trials by interested professionals. Those who favour labour and birth in water say that its benefits include freedom of movement, effective pain relief, acceleration of labour, lowering of blood pressure, less perineal trauma, less interventions of most kinds, and a gentler entry into the world for the baby. Much of this is borne out by available research.

Critics say that there is an increased risk of infection for mother, baby and midwife, that water inhibits contractions, that it increases the risk of perineal trauma, that it increases risk of post-partum haemorrhage and makes birth a traumatic experience for the baby. None of this is proven by any known scientific evidence.

'Water birth' should not necessarily be viewed as a superior form of birth. It is simply another variation. Many mothers do not wish nor are suitable (for instance if they are in premature labour, before 37 weeks) for birth in water. But this does not mean that their births cannot be calm, empowering, wonderful experiences.

Water Birth Safety

At the First Annual Waterbirth Conference at Wembley Stadium in 1995, an unofficial sign on the wall read, 'Water birth is unsafe – for obstetricians'. Obstetricians in particular seem to feel threatened by the 'do it yourself' nature of many water births, and by the fact that a woman in water can labour, and even give birth, quite happily without their help.

While there is no evidence to show that labouring or giving birth in water is unsafe, two crucial issues have emerged. Problems can occur when the water is too hot or the baby is left under water for extended periods of time after delivery. Labouring in very hot water over several hours has been linked with hyperthermia (over-heating), which is a possible cause of brain damage to or the death of the baby. Also, a few babies have died as a result of being held under water by naïve people who felt that a longer period under water would ease the transition from water to air for the baby.

Making water labour or birth safe is largely a matter of common sense. The water should be blood temperature for delivery, and only a few degrees either side of that during labour. Emerging from the mother's body *is* the baby's transition from water to air. While there have been reports of babies surviving unharmed for a minute or two under water, the *only* safe advice is to bring the baby to the surface calmly as soon as it is born. Parents and attendants must curb their tendency to control the process of birth, even when using essentially harmless, 'alternative' methods.

Looking Ahead – Birth Options

To date we have to rely on small studies only, but the data is remarkably consistent. A survey of water labour and birth in England and Wales in 1993 showed that a total of 8,255 women laboured in water but got out for birth, and 4,494 gave birth in the water. In total, 12 babies died after their mothers laboured or gave birth in water, but none of these cases was reported to be directly related to water birth or labour. A further 51 babies did have some form of morbidity (illness) such as breathing difficulties or infection. It is not clear, because of the retrospective nature of the study, how many of these were directly related to water labour or birth.[37]

The safety of this kind of birth may not have so much to do with the water as it does with what the water stands for. In simple terms, a mother who is labouring or birthing in water is much harder to interfere with. Enclosed within the boundaries of the pool, she is more protected and autonomous. She can't easily be fitted with monitoring belts or jabbed with needles. She is protected. The low rates of intervention for women who labour and give birth in water may be directly related to this. It may also be that doctors and midwives, in the presence of a woman labouring in a secure and self-possessed manner, are able to change their perceptions and behaviour accordingly.

There seems to be some indication that, especially for first-time mothers – the group which is on the receiving end of most obstetric interventions – labouring in water may reduce levels of pain to such a degree that they use significantly less pain-relieving drugs. In one group of first-time mothers labouring in water, only 24 per cent used pain-relieving drugs, compared to 50 per cent of those labouring out of water.[38]

Similarly, another study showed that labouring in water reduces the tendency for attendants to induce labour or perform episiotomies. In this study, none of the water-birth mothers had episiotomies, as opposed to 27 per cent of first-time mothers and 8 per cent of second-time or more mothers in the bed-birth group.[39]

Interestingly, the same study found that only 16 per cent of the water-birth mothers heard about the option of using a birthing pool from their midwife – 39 per cent first heard about it through the media. This seems to be the same everywhere: Hospitals have birthing pools, but do not seem to encourage women to use them.

It appears that, once in the water and given the choice, about half of the women stay there whether they originally intended to or not. Women find they are so relaxed in the water they are reluctant to emerge for the birth. Realistically speaking there is no reason why they should, and this makes some practitioners nervous. Some women are asked to sign a form swearing that they will get out of the water to give birth. This is another form of blackmail and has no standing in law. Even if a mother does agree to sign, she is under no obligation to get out of the water if she changes her mind during labour. Possession of a mother's signature on a piece of paper does not protect an unskilled or negligent practitioner should anything go wrong. If a woman refuses to get out of the water, it is up to the midwife to carry out her professional duty – to deliver a healthy baby and look after the mother's safety – to the best of her ability.

In the summer of 1994 the United Kingdom Central Council for Nursing, Midwifery and Health Visiting (UKCC) made their position on water birth clear. They recognized that '... waterbirth is preferred by some women as their chosen method for delivery of their babies. Waterbirth should, therefore, be viewed as an alternative method of care and management in labour and as one which must, therefore, fall within the duty of care and normal sphere of the practice of a midwife.'[40]

All midwives are required, by their professional code of conduct, to be responsible for keeping their skills up to date and to acquire new skills as and when their job demands. If a practitioner is truly out of her depth, then it is up to the hospital to provide someone who has more experience. Labour and birth in water, like birth in general, is only unsafe in unskilled hands.

For the Baby's Good?

For the duration of your ante-natal care and particularly when you are giving birth you might hear phrases such as 'It's the best thing for your baby,' 'Your baby will benefit from this' or 'You owe it to your baby.' The unborn baby is now a silent but powerful influence on just about everything which is done to and for a mother. Ultrasound technology has made it possible for us to see the baby before it's born, making it seem more 'real'. But, in spite of this visual breakthrough, a baby *in utero* is, in many ways, a fantasy creature and, as such, we are all free to project our own prejudices and fears onto it and to use it as we like to twist an argument in our favour.

The 'good of the baby' is often invoked in arguments by doctors and mothers as the best possible reason for doing or not doing something. A doctor who can't make a mother 'see sense' for her own sake may hit her in her soft spot with the idea of doing it 'for the sake of your baby'. A mother who can't speak up for herself or who feels she isn't being heard may use the idea of the baby's welfare simply as a manipulative tool for getting what she wants. Sometimes 'concern for the baby' shadows a concern for being right and being seen to be in control of the situation.

The baby's welfare and the baby's rights are a tricky and emotive subject. While no one would deny that a mother has a moral obligation to look after her unborn child – and the vast majority of mothers take this obligation very seriously – a baby *in utero* has no standing in UK law. It is generally accepted that a mother will always act in the best interests of her baby, and as a result there have been no moves to legislate on its behalf.

What this means is that a fetus has no 'right' to treatment and a mother cannot be forced to do anything for her baby which she simply does not want to, which she feels will do more harm than good, or to which she has a religious or moral objection to. According to the Medical Defence Union, a doctor's first obligation is to the mother. Given a choice between treatment which will help the mother and treatment which will help her unborn child, the doctor must first act to help the mother.[41]

This premise has been severely tested both here and in the United States recently, where a spate of attempted (and in some cases successful) enforced caesarean operations have been the subject of widespread criticism by legal and consumer advocates alike. Barrister Barbara Hewson reminds us that a competent adult cannot even have a blood test without giving consent, and yet grown women here and in the US have been forced, sometimes dragged, kicking, screaming and handcuffed, to the operating table 'for the good of the baby'. She believes, rightly, that 'allowing obstetricians to cut open women's bodies against their will as a means of saving their fetus, is open to powerful moral and legal objections,'[42] and furthermore that:

> There is an additional case for saying that denying pregnant women the same rights as other adults, competent patients to refuse surgery, constitutes unlawful sex discrimination on pregnancy grounds by a service provider, contrary to section 29, Sex Discrimination Act 1975 ... an obstetrician who threatens a privately paying patient with compulsory surgery might be made the subject of a formal complaint of consumer abuse to the Office of Fair Trading under section 34, Fair Trading Act 1973.[43]

In this debate, the Royal College of Obstetricians and Gynaecologists also came down on the side of the mother, albeit with the security of knowing that, having discharged their professional duty to the best of their ability, should 'ill nevertheless befall' they were legally protected. It concluded that 'obstetricians must respect the woman's legal liberty to ignore or reject professional advice, even to her own detriment and that of her fetus.'[44]

Interestingly, in the debate about the baby's needs and the baby's good we often forget about the true and important role which the baby does play, namely in labour. Labour isn't just something which mothers and doctors go through in order to help the baby out. The baby is an active partner in the whole process as well. It is the baby's readiness to be born in the first place which triggers the hormonal changes in the mother which in turn prepare her body for labour. Over the last few weeks of pregnancy a woman's body changes rapidly. Her cervix softens, the muscles and ligaments in the pelvis relax. Inside, the baby may be putting on a final growth spurt and, particularly in first pregnancies, it is common for the baby's head to settle, or 'engage' in the pelvis during this time. Physically and emotionally both mother and baby may be more 'settled'. The baby may seem to move less and the mother may find herself becoming more introspective.

Once labour has started, the baby again takes an active role. Its head pressing down, assisted by its own weight and the force of gravity (if the mother is able to be in an upright position) help in the process of opening out the cervix. Working with the force of the contractions, the baby will wiggle its way into the best position to pass through the birth canal. Some mothers find that their babies kick a lot during labour. You may be surprised to feel your baby using the top of your uterus as a brace to push against. This is the response of a healthy baby who wants to be born. Unfortunately, this response can be dulled by the use of drugs, which may bring welcome pain relief but can impede progress for both mother and baby.

Pregnancy and birth are journeys which mother and baby take together. Given the chance, your baby, who has been your constant companion for nine months, can end up being your single biggest help during the hours of labour.

2
Meeting the 'Experts'

There is no other time in a woman's life when she will meet so many people, over such a short period of time, who may claim to know more about her than she does. In this respect pregnancy can prove to be very frustrating. General practitioners, midwives, consultant obstetricians, radiographers, paediatricians, health visitors and students of every description advise, poke, prod and discuss her body and her baby, often as if she weren't really there or aware of what was happening to her at all.

Be that as it may, expectant mothers are very sensitive. Even those who are ordinarily totally in command of themselves are very impressionable and receptive to what is said and done around them. It can hardly be stressed enough – the people who surround you during your pregnancy have an exceptionally strong influence on your well-being. The manner and extent to which different practitioners participate in your ante-natal care, and in your labour, can shape the experience, making it either satisfying and fulfilling or disappointing and, in some cases, deeply distressing and disempowering. That is why it's important to choose carefully.

In the light of this, learning something about doctors' and midwives' roles – what they can and can't do, what their limitations and areas of expertise are, and where their loyalties lie, becomes more than just an intellectual exercise. It becomes the key to restoring the balance of power between women and those who care for them. This, in turn, can make it very much easier for women to exercise their right of choice confidently throughout pregnancy, birth and beyond.

Realistically speaking, our choices are, to a large extent, limited by the influence of more general policies (made by the government, health authorities, and Trusts) for health care and personnel. Forces beyond our control decide who should provide care and what kind of care it should be. This presents certain problems, especially when it comes to maternity care. As Marsden Wagner of the World Health Organization points out:

> First, in many countries these policies are not determined mainly through careful, rational assessment of what is needed and what resources are available. Other less rational factors predominate, such as the influence of the most powerful groups in the health sector, special interest groups (including commercial interests) and particular people.
>
> Second, even if policies on health care and personnel are based on rational assessment, it is inappropriate to apply the principles used for assessing general health care needs to maternity care needs. The birth process creates needs different from any other that the health care system must meet.[1]

The assertion of women's rights as consumers of health care with unique needs and as experts about their bodies and their babies puts many professionals on the defensive. Few of us feel comfortable with the image of health practitioners and mothers on opposing sides. Neither are we at ease with the juxtaposition of 'war' words such as 'control', 'battle', 'struggle' and 'power' next to words like 'baby', 'mother' and 'birth'. But the truth is that

Meeting the 'Experts'

many of the policies and routine practices in maternity care today are based on 'power' – who has it, who hasn't, who's going to get it and especially who's going to use it and how. As a result many practitioners are desperately trying to hold on to what little power they feel they have left. Consultants and GPs are afraid of losing out to, and being challenged by, the expertise of mothers and the professional autonomy of midwives. Midwives are afraid of losing out to consultants, general practitioners and mothers, and mothers usually end up somewhere at the bottom of the heap, temporary visitors in the hospital power structure.

Mothers and Doctors

Relationships between women and their doctors also take on an extra dynamic during pregnancy. Up until that point a woman has probably been used to managing her own health and that of her family, and possibly even that of her friends, alone, and often with great skill.

People often look to the women in their lives as the first point of contact when they are ill. Many illnesses never get to the doctor at all because they are dealt with by women, at home. The fact that most of these illnesses are minor does not make the job of tending to them any less skilled. As Helen Roberts points out:

> Women may not be taking out the appendix, treating the duodenal ulcer, stripping the varicose veins, but they are doing the bulk of health care in our society, the bulk of preventative work and, possibly, even giving the bulk of advice. This advice is so much a part of our everyday lives that we hardly even see it as advice: 'Don't eat that Sam, it will rot your teeth', 'Try rubbing in some oil to get rid of his cradle cap', 'A dry biscuit in the morning first thing when I was pregnant used to stop me feeling so sick. Why not try that?' There is, though, a real cold war over women as producers of knowledge about health care. Doctors have long warned us about going to another woman for advice ...[2]

Curiously, though, when women need professional help and go to doctors for advice they are not always given what they need. Often they are given reassurance rather than information, or they are made to feel like little girls who are taking up the doctor's valuable time with trivial worries instead of grown women asking legitimate questions. A paradoxical attitude from a profession so keen to preserve its image as 'expert'!

Of course, what is said here (and throughout this book) about doctors can also apply to midwives, health visitors and all other practitioners, whose training emphasizes their role as experts who are in charge of a 'situation', rather than as partners in a unique, natural process.

The relationship between women and doctors is further complicated during pregnancy by the presence of an unseen third party, the baby. The concept of the baby as a patient is relatively new.[3] It evolved when X-rays, and later ultrasound techniques, enabled doctors to see a child *in utero* for the first time. The fact that the baby is now *seen*, rather than *imagined*, to be a living thing makes differences of opinion between mothers and doctors potentially quite significant, giving rise as it does to conflicting sets of emotions and values.

For instance, while most women might assume that a doctor would only advise a caesarean with the safety of mother and baby uppermost in his mind, research shows that fear of litigation is the primary reason why doctors perform this operation.[4] Equally, a doctor's enthusiasm for ante-natal testing, or offering a termination as a 'solution' to a baby with abnormalities, may come from pressure put upon him to keep hospital statistics for abnormalities below the national average, rather than a concern for mother and baby. A mother may have other, more complex and personal reasons for choosing tests or a termination.

While some medical advances have certainly helped in the management of complicated pregnancies, for the majority of women with straightforward pregnancies and healthy babies these advances have meant simply that doctors now have power over two lives instead of one. For a woman to be involved in making decisions about her care, practitioners must relinquish some of their power. It is a concept which can be deeply threatening to all practitioners, particularly obstetricians, of both sexes.

Some practitioners have even less rational reasons for the things they say and do. A doctor who disapproves of labouring in water or home birth may simply be trying to hide the fact that he has no professional or personal experience, or indeed any training, in these areas. A midwife who tells a moaning woman in labour not to make so much noise may be uncomfortable with her own sexuality and thus the sexual noises a labouring woman makes. A health visitor who encourages a mother to bottle-feed an infant may have 'failed' to breastfeed herself, and thus may have difficulty accepting that other women can 'succeed'.

In addition, few of us realize how traumatic medical education can be. Not only are the hours long and the institutional stressors enormous, but in most medical education, particularly in obstetrics and gynaecology, the focus is always on the abnormal, the times when things go wrong. Most practitioners are trained to act, not to observe. So when they are called upon to exercise the kind of expectant watchfulness appropriate to maternity care, they feel anxious, disempowered and underemployed. The damage which the system inflicts on its practitioners, and the way this is passed on to mothers, cannot be ignored or taken lightly.

As a result of their education and experience, each of the three main types of practitioner with whom a woman will come into contact – midwife, GP and obstetrician – will have a very different perspective on birth. For the midwife, birth is a personal and social event; for the obstetrician it is a medical one; for the general practitioner it falls somewhere in between.

What's more, birth can look very different placed in different contexts. A hi-tech atmosphere, now so common in hospital, breeds fear of the process, particularly in doctors, and a feeling of being involved in a medical emergency which, in turn, necessitates the current trend of placing upper time-limits on each stage of labour and the early and copious application of interventions.

Every Woman's BirthRights

A medically-orientated practitioner stepping out of this environment into a smaller GP- or midwife-led unit might feel fearful about the lack of intervention and the tendency to 'allow' labour to go on longer before interfering. The same practitioner might feel terrified watching a woman give birth at home, where she is totally in control, at her own pace, in her own way. As a result there is as much conflict between people within the maternity services as there is among those who observe and campaign for change from the outside.

It is certainly relevant to be aware of these power issues, as long as you are also aware that you are not obliged to become too entangled in them. You do not need to feel sorry for the midwife who has a busy clinic or who has been up all night, the doctor who has just presided over a disastrous birth, the overworked SHO (Senior House Officer) or health visitor who can't give you the time or information you need. It is not your job to understand or listen to problems which, after all, come with the job.

When considering the range of professionals who can attend you during pregnancy and birth, it may also be helpful to remember that whether you are using the NHS or private healthcare you are paying for a service, either directly or through your taxes. Healthcare practitioners are there to attend you, to advise and discuss methods and procedures with you, not to lay down the law. Ironically there is very little law governing the actions of doctors and the rights of patients. But what little there is, is very clear. No practitioner has the power to force you to do anything against your will. Nor can you be given any treatment without your consent. To do so constitutes an assault under common law for which the doctor or midwife can be prosecuted.

The information which follows has been compiled with all these issues in mind. It takes into account the social, professional, legal and ethical agendas which make a mother's choice of practitioner so crucial. Remember that if you find that you are unsatisfied with the practitioner(s) you have chosen or (as is much more common) been allocated, you have the right to change to another carer *at any time* during your pregnancy or

Meeting the 'Experts'

even during labour (though few women can realistically be expected to feel secure enough to exercise the latter option). You do not need anybody's permission to change your mind. It is entirely your decision.

General Practitioners

Your GP is probably the first person you will encounter when you think or know you are pregnant. GPs are involved to a greater or lesser extent in the ante-natal care of around 98 per cent of British women. This care can amount to an initial consultation, some or all of a woman's ante-natal care and, in rare circumstances (less than 6 per cent of births), attending some or all of her labour. He may also provide some form of postnatal care and support.

Some women feel comfortable with the fact that their own GP is a familiar face who already knows their medical history. Theoretically he is also someone who can view their pregnancy in the fuller emotional, psychological and social context of their lives. GPs have the advantage of being based in the local community, of being on call 24 hours a day if needed and of being generalists able to provide the kind of simple care appropriate for the majority of women with healthy pregnancies. Occasionally they care for families not just for years but for generations. Women receiving GP care may feel they are being treated more like individuals and, if they are lucky, will feel that their doctor is taking more time over them.

But there are problems with the current standard of GP care in the UK. First, while any GP can provide ante-natal care, not all have the qualifications to do so. It is important that you establish your GPs qualifications right from the start. Many women feel it is impudent to ask what a doctor's qualifications are. After all, he went to medical school for all those years. Some doctors may reply, 'My qualifications? I've been doing this job for 20 years – those are my qualifications.' This is not an answer. Length of service is no guarantee of good practice. There are GPs out there who have been routinely making the same mistakes for years.

Some doctors, when asked, may deflect the question back at you and ask you what your qualifications are. The answer is simple: you're a woman and you can read. You and your baby deserve the best care possible, and establishing your doctor's qualifications is a first step towards getting that care.

If your GP is on the 'obstetrics list' it is an indication that he has received some special training in obstetrics. If he's not on the list, find one who is. Doctors who are not on the obstetrics list should not be looking after pregnant women. If your GP will not help you do this, you can go to your post office or public library, or contact your local Family Health Services Authority (FHSA) to find out for yourself which GPs in your area are on the list. You can then ask to be referred, or refer yourself, to the doctor of your choice. Even if your GP is on the obstetrics list, you have the right to transfer to another doctor in your area if you feel you would receive better care.

Having said that, the obstetrics list is not an automatic guarantee of a higher standard of care. At the moment there are no national criteria for inclusion on the list. This is a scandal, because criteria, which are set by individual FHSAs, can vary enormously. Some associations only require a practitioner to have completed a six-month residency on an obstetrics ward, as part of his general practitioner training (something which most GPs have done, albeit 20 years ago). Others require more substantial and recent training.

Once a doctor is on the obstetrics list he cannot be removed from it, nor will he be required to keep his training up to date – an issue which is causing great concern among professional and lay groups alike. It's a sad, but very real possibility, that when you walk into a doctor's surgery armed with all the latest information about pregnancy and childbirth, you may actually know more than he does about certain things!

General practitioners who have the letters DRCOG after their name have taken a diploma in obstetrics and gynaecology from the Royal College of Obstetricians and Gynaecologists, with a view to providing ante-natal care for women with normal

Meeting the 'Experts'

pregnancies and even attending births in GP units. You are on somewhat safer ground with a practitioner with these qualifications (even if they were gained some years ago), as there is at least a chance that this is a person who is enthusiastic about and interested in childbirth rather than one who has simply applied for inclusion on the obstetrics list because it brings more money into the practice.

Be mindful, though, that a GP who has trained in obstetrics may inevitably carry his own special prejudices. He will have trained in a large teaching hospital under the guidance of a consultant obstetrician and will have learned primarily about all the things that can go wrong during pregnancy and birth. He will have learned, wrongly, to think of pregnancy as an illness. As a result, he may employ practices and routines which might be ineffective or inappropriate for a healthy expectant mother. This is because the roles of the GP and specialist are essentially different. A GP is a generalist whose role is to oversee the 'normal' and to identify those deviations from the normal that require referral to a specialist. An obstetrician's job is primarily to identify and manage the abnormal.

Advantages:

* Your own GP is a familiar face throughout your pregnancy. At the moment GPs probably provide the greatest continuity of care for pregnant women.

* If you are worried that something is wrong, and you can't get to the surgery, your GP can attend you at home and can, theoretically, provide 24-hour care.

* GP clinics are usually smaller and within the local area.

* GPs are usually well placed to provide the sort of generalized, low-intervention care which the majority of women with healthy pregnancies require.

Disadvantages:

* Some GPs are reluctant to refer women to, or share care with, a midwife. Occasionally this reluctance has more to do with money than with care – GPs do not get paid as much for shared care schemes.

* Your GP is not required to keep his training up to date, so his knowledge can be out of date.

* In some circumstances GP care can be as authoritarian and pathologically-orientated as consultant care.

* The majority of GPs are men – which may make it hard for them to view pregnancy with the same sort of empathy that you might receive from another woman.

* If your relationship with your GP is no good, your ante-natal care could turn out to be a depressing experience.

* If you request a transfer to another GP for your ante-natal care, your own GP may feel personally insulted and strike you off (and, in some cases, other members of your family) off his list – even though the RCOG and the RCGP have agreed that this is poor behaviour and totally unnecessary. However, once you have registered with a GP for *ante-natal care* you cannot be struck off without your consent or without the GP first applying to the FHSA for permission (he will need a good reason). If he does not do this he is in breach of his contract of employment with the FHSA.

* Few GPs support home births.

* If you have shared care with a GP and a midwife, neither of whom is very skilled, they can miss potential problems. Some women end up with very poor care indeed.

Meeting the 'Experts'

Midwives

Midwives are specialists in normal pregnancy and birth. We are extremely lucky in the UK to have a system of midwifery care which remains more or less intact. In parts of the US and Canada, and even in some other European countries, the practice of midwifery is either struggling to survive or has been outlawed altogether. There is little doubt that a midwife is the best person to oversee a normal pregnancy and birth. Midwives are trained professionals and they are autonomous and able to exercise their own clinical judgement independent of doctors. You can book a midwife for your total care whether you intend to have your baby in hospital or at home. You don't need your GP's permission to do this, and you don't have to report to or confirm your pregnancy with him beforehand. To book midwifery care, simply contact the Supervisor of Midwives at your local hospital.

The great majority of midwives are dedicated, enthusiastic, conscientious women who are also, for the most part, more in tune with the concepts of informed choice and birth as a normal physiological (without technological interventions) experience. They are the only practitioners whose training is based solely on the care and well-being of mothers and their babies.

Midwifery has been practised here and throughout Europe and the rest of the world for centuries. Historically a midwife would have been an older woman who had children of her own as well as wide experience of attending births in the community. A female companion has long been accepted as the best kind of 'medicine' for another woman in labour, and even today researchers find that outcomes improve if a *doula* (a 'trained' female birth partner) is present.[5] In one study, the presence of a doula was shown to cut the average length of labour, from admission to delivery, by half (from 19.3 hours to 8.8 hours!).[6]

Midwives today have a different profile. In many ways the profession has become task-centred rather than woman-centred, involving a number of peripheral routine tasks and duties which can get in the way of a midwife's first duty – to support women.

Also, today there are a number of midwives who are young and/or have no children of their own; indeed there are some who have no desire to have children of their own. No matter how many births they attend, some may never develop a deep understanding of the impact which having a baby has on women, personally and socially. This can be a great disadvantage for the mothers in their care.

In addition, there are two different types of midwives coming from two distinctly different educational backgrounds, both trading under the name of 'Midwife'. First there are those who trained initially as nurses and then decided to take up midwifery training later. They come from a medical background and tend to bring this ethos to their practice. Then there are midwives who come from lay backgrounds into what is known as 'direct entry' training programmes. Some of these women are older, they have experience of life outside the medical world, they may have children and are often very positive about the process and potential of birth. Obviously these are generalizations, but the point is that you may benefit from asking your midwife a few questions about her beliefs and her background.

Midwives work in a wide range of settings, such as hospitals, in local community clinics, and in private practices which take them directly into women's homes. Hospital-based midwives can be very different from those based in the community, and these women in turn can be very different from independent midwives who practise privately.

In the hospital setting midwives wear uniforms which make them almost indistinguishable from nurses – though the two professions are quite different. Often they become distracted by the routines of administration: they make appointments, check women's weight, check blood pressure, assess urine samples, oversee vaginal examinations performed by doctors and keep records and charts up to date. For many their day-to-day job is more like that of a secretary than a health practitioner, and there are those who are never given, and never ask for, more responsibility than this.

Hospital midwives are expected to follow hospital policy, which is set by the consultant obstetrician. Unfortunately, hospital policies often place midwives in direct conflict with the codes of conduct which govern their own profession by requiring their first loyalty to be to their employers rather than to the women in their care. Some spirited midwives choose to fight this compromising state of affairs from within. They join groups such as the Association of Radical Midwives (ARM) and support each other in the uphill struggle to make doctors see how damaging some of their policies are. Unfortunately there are relatively few rewards for speaking out. Mothers may love these individuals, but a midwife can find herself in danger of losing her job if she bucks the system too often. Other midwives opt out altogether and seek to practise independently – a choice which is currently being threatened by the increasingly high costs of setting up and of indemnity insurance.

In some areas the only way for a woman to be attended in labour by a midwife she knows is for her to book a Domino delivery (*see page 11*), otherwise she will be attended by whoever is on duty. However, in order to meet a recent government mandate which states that 'within 5 years' time 75 per cent of women should be cared for in labour by a midwife whom they have come to know during pregnancy,'[7] many hospitals have begun to implement practices such as team midwifery and group practices. Both involve small teams of midwives, usually no more than six, either working from the hospital or in local clinics. The midwives take on a defined caseload and give total care to the women registered with them. Some midwives see this kind of change in working practice as a dynamic and positive step for midwifery and for mothers.

For others, who are comfortable with the hospital routine, this mandate is very threatening because it asks them to take on responsibilities for continuity of care and for being a named midwife (and therefore totally responsible for a woman's care throughout her pregnancy and labour) rather than simply processing her through the system. Some individuals have neither the education, the experience, the skill nor the inclination to do this.

Do not underestimate the influence of your midwife on your pregnancy and labour. A quiet, confident, 'together' midwife will be a woman's anchor in labour and a buffer against the often senseless hospital routines imposed on mothers during pregnancy. Under midwifery care mothers are likely to have significantly less interventions in labour. Most significant is the lower rate of electronic fetal monitoring – the introduction of which is known to lead to a cascade of other, possibly unnecessary, interventions.[8] In addition, mothers are likely to have stronger feelings of empowerment and satisfaction after birth if they have been cared for by a midwife.

But the reverse can also be true. A midwife who is herself very afraid of birth or who is uneasy with her own sexuality or who feels disempowered professionally can unwittingly turn an otherwise straightforward labour into a parade of interventions in the name of rescuing the mother and/or baby from distress.

If you find a midwife who is really on your side and who is genuinely enthusiastic about childbirth – hang on to her. At the moment, midwifery in Britain is truly on the brink. In addition to all the power struggles and the reorganization of methods of care, the whole system of midwifery training is systematically being taken out of hospitals and into centres of higher education where theoretical and academic achievements take priority over hands-on experience. Midwifery is not an academic exercise but an essential service for pregnant women and mothers. There is an urgent need for midwives and mothers to value and support each other. If they don't there is a real and persistent danger that the whole system of maternity care will fall rapidly into medical hands and the whole concept of woman-centred care will simply disappear.

If you find a midwife whom you find unenthusiastic, regimented and negative about your plans for your pregnancy and birth, dismiss her as soon as possible. You can do this by contacting the Supervisor of Midwives and asking for a different

Meeting the 'Experts'

midwife. Do not wait until late in your pregnancy, when a change in carer can cause a great deal of emotional (as well as clinical) upheaval.

Advantages:

* Midwives are specialists in 'normal' pregnancy and childbirth. Close to 90 per cent of pregnant women are normal and healthy and require no special treatments or interventions.

* Midwives are the only practitioners who are required to keep their training up to date. They must apply for re-registration each year and show that they have read the research and attended approved courses and seminars to help keep their skills up to date.

* Midwives can provide continuity of care, particularly in areas where there is sensitively organized and implemented team midwifery or group practice.

* Midwives are able to give total care, including access to diagnostic tests and hospital beds. You can book your care with a midwife without having to go through a GP or ask his permission.

* The majority of midwives are women, and many mothers feel more comfortable with a woman attending them.

* Most midwives put the mother's needs first – even when they are governed by conflicting sets of guidelines from their own professional bodies and the hospitals they work in.

Disadvantages:

* Some midwives who come from a nursing background tend to think of mothers as patients and try to actively manage their pregnancies and labours.

* Midwifery training does not place enough emphasis on counselling skills and on the two-way nature of the midwife/mother relationship. Some midwives carry personal/emotional baggage into their jobs, which means that the way they advise women about things such as nutrition, methods of pain relief and breastfeeding can be based more on prejudice than medical fact.

* A midwife who has a negative view of pregnancy and childbirth can quickly breed fear and a sense of failure in a mother, making it difficult for the mother to have a normal physiological birth and a sense of fulfilment from the experience.

Independent Midwives
Many women find the choice of an independent midwife is often the best way to avoid a technologically-managed birth, and this can help them to gain confidence in their own bodies, in the process of birth and their ability to cope with whatever comes. Private midwifery care has several advantages, not just for individual women but also for the continued positive perception of the midwifery profession.

Independent midwives can provide a total service, including ante-natal, birth and postnatal care. Midwives who have chosen to work in the private sector usually have some experience of working within the NHS as well. Often they have decided to work independently because they have become very dissatisfied with the restrictions and routines within the hospital hierarchy. Many are fiercely loyal to the idea of mother-centred care and resist the idea of the technological imperative of modern birth.

Meeting the 'Experts'

The cost of private midwifery care is not usually covered in health insurance policies. However, many independent midwives offer schemes which will allow a mother to spread payments over the period of ante-natal care and beyond if necessary.

Independent midwives usually work in small teams or group practices. Early in your ante-natal care you will be given the chance to choose which midwife you want as your lead professional, and you will be given the opportunity to get to know all the other midwives in the group as well. Ante-natal appointments will be in your own home, and some midwives will even visit you in your office or place of work, if necessary. Independent midwives carry everything necessary to assist a safe birth at home. They also carry some pain-relieving drugs (gas, air and pethidine) and resuscitation equipment.

While most independent midwives carry insurance against accidents and litigation, some find the high cost of this insurance crippling and have elected to practise without it. You should find out beforehand if your midwife is insured. The risk of an accident is very small, but some parents may still feel better knowing they are with a midwife who is insured. The vast majority of independent midwives are consummate and enthusiastic professionals. Inevitably, though, there are some who are not so conscientious. Always ask questions and make sure you feel comfortable with any potential carer.

You can get a list of the independent midwives in your area by contacting the Independent Midwives Association (*see Appendix C for address*).

Advantages:

* Private midwives are empowered to give you total care, including access to hospital beds, tests and equipment in an emergency or if they think you need extra help, as well as arranging GP cover if they feel it is needed.

- In some areas, employing a private midwife may actually be the only way to achieve a home birth without a continuous battle.

- Most independent midwives will help you to spread the cost of their services over the period of your ante-natal care and beyond if necessary.

- Independent midwives can attend you in hospital or at home – the choice is yours.

Disadvantages:

- A small number of independent midwives are forced to practise without insurance. You may find this unacceptable.

- Apart from the cost, which can be anything from £2,000 upwards and may be prohibitive to most people, there are few disadvantages to private midwifery care.

- Independent midwives attending births at home do not have access to the same range of emergency equipment as those working in hospitals.

- Although it is rare, there are a few independent midwives of questionable skill and expertise.

Obstetricians

Since so few women actually have complicated pregnancies, obstetrics should be a very small speciality. Yet the obstetrician is one of the most powerful players in the world of pregnancy and childbirth. In simple terms, obstetricians are specialists in abnormality. The whole focus of their training (indeed the entire history of the profession) is based on pursuing, diagnosing and treating reproductive pathology (abnormality and disease).

Meeting the 'Experts'

The consultant obstetrician works in the hospital and is responsible for setting the policy for his 'team' – midwives, obstetric nurses, radiologists, neonatologists, anaesthetists, etc. He trains his students according to what he knows (and sometimes that knowledge is quite outdated, because professional guidelines do not require obstetricians to keep their training up to date). One survey in 1994, designed to determine the awareness among obstetricians of a comprehensive, well-respected and widely available database of evidence-based obstetric information known as the Cochrane Collaboration Pregnancy and Childbirth Database, produced grim results.[9] Only 29 per cent of obstetric consultants could define what the database was, and some 72 per cent of the obstetric units questioned did not have access to it. The justification for not using the database revealed astonishing arrogance and some very entrenched attitudes. Among them: 'We are a teaching hospital so we don't need to know what everyone else is doing' and 'Obstetrics is an art, not a science.'

The implication here is important. Even when faced with research findings which demonstrate that their firmly-held beliefs about what is best for pregnant or birthing women are wrong, few obstetricians are willing to modify their views or their practice.

Motivating consultants to keep up to date is now recognized as a real problem.[10] Although the Royal College of Obstetricians and Gynaecologists does operate a 'points system' to encourage doctors to pursue further education and training (members can acquire up to 500 'brownie' points and a piece of paper for their office walls for going to approved classes and seminars), even this is not compulsory and it's hard to see much enthusiasm among members for the idea.

The choice of a private obstetrician does not necessarily guarantee a better standard of care. When you choose an obstetrician, whether he is in the public or private sector, you are also choosing the institution in which he practises. Obstetricians practise in hospitals, not because hospitals provide a safer environment for birth, but because they are now the only places big enough to hold the technology which has become so instrumental to the profession. Obstetric technology can be seductive. In some cases it can be appealing enough to make a doctor forget the primary tenet of the Hippocratic oath: 'First, do nothing.'

As recently as 40 years ago, undergraduate medical schools were still preaching the doctrine of 'masterly inactivity', waiting for the process of birth to complete itself naturally. But as Marjorie Tew observes:

> When after 1950 ... obstetricians became more confident to use interventions at their disposal, they increasingly abandoned the philosophy of restraint. They redefined normality in pregnancy and labour to justify the widespread practice of antenatal, intranatal and postnatal interventions, so that the need, as they perceived it, for most births to take place in hospital became inevitable. And since obstetricians, despite their vaunted skills, could never predict with accuracy when a complication would arise, the sensible precaution was to take every step to ensure that all births should take place in their kind of hospital.[11]

As recently as the mid-1980s some members of the obstetric profession even campaigned to make hospital birth compulsory and home birth illegal. This came to nothing, perhaps because the public outcry at such a move would only serve to undermine the enormous, and somewhat spurious, public and professional confidence which obstetricians have worked so long to maintain.

Obstetricians historically regard themselves as the Rolls Royce of maternity care, and all other practitioners as Reliant Robins; for the most part the public has gone along with this view. Unfortunately this widespread confidence in the miracle of obstetrics has led to a corresponding undermining of mothers' confidence in their own bodies and reproductive skill, as well as eroding the confidence of midwives and general practitioners in the importance of their role as overseers of the vast majority of normal, healthy pregnant women.

Meeting the 'Experts'

Not all obstetricians, however, are so self-important. A small number ply their trade in a more appropriate manner, restricting their involvement to women with complicated pregnancies and being actively enthusiastic about the role of their colleagues in midwifery and general practice. These individuals know that acknowledging the ability and expertise of midwives and GPs, and the uncomplicated nature of most pregnancies, means they can devote more time and care to those women who genuinely need their skills.

If you want or need to be cared for by an obstetrician, you will be referred to one by your GP (although there are calls for re-thinking this system and giving people direct access to consultants and specialists in all areas of medical practice). What usually happens is your GP will refer you to whichever consultant he has the best relationship with. You don't have to accept this. If you know which consultant you want, you can ask to be referred to him. If you don't, you do not have to agree to be booked under anyone until you have found out something about the way he practises. You can do this by speaking to other mothers who have had babies in that hospital or by writing to your Community Health Council or to the hospital administrator and asking for information on a specific consultant's policies (rates of interventions, operative deliveries, inductions, etc.). Your GP may urge you to hurry up and decide, but you are not obliged to adhere to any particular time limit.

Advantages:

* There are no proven medical advantages to obstetric care for a healthy woman with a healthy baby.

* Women who feel especially worried or anxious about being pregnant may feel more reassured knowing that a specialist is on hand 'just to be on the safe side'. However, it should be noted that under midwife care, should something go wrong the obstetrician would be called in

immediately and must attend. Under GP care a woman who develops complications will be referred to a specialist consultant.

Disadvantages:

* Obstetricians are specialists in abnormality – many have never seen a normal physiological birth. Their own criteria for what is 'normal' is very narrow and predisposes them to intervene earlier and with less clinical indication than other practitioners.

* Obstetric interventions can create complications where there are none. For instance, the seemingly simple act of rupturing a woman's membranes (so her waters break) can lead to a 'cascade of interventions' which ends with an emergency caesarean.

* The obstetrician, unlike the GP, knows nothing about you and will not be able to view your pregnancy in its wider emotional, social and psychological context.

* Don't be fooled by a white coat. Many obstetricians have other priorities such as private practices and teaching duties, which mean that you will rarely see the consultant with whom you are registered. Instead you will generally be attended by an SHO (Senior House Officer), a medical student doing his residency in the obstetrics ward. This, of course, makes a nonsense of the idea of getting specialist care, as not all the SHOs in a maternity ward have an interest in obstetrics or will go on to be obstetricians themselves.

* If you find you are not confident about the procedure, it can be more difficult to switch from obstetric care to midwifery care than vice versa.

* Consultant obstetricians rarely inform women about their maternity care options or acknowledge women's right to choose.

* Obstetricians do not always behave in the consistent and scientific manner which we assume they do. They are not obliged to keep their training up to date and many are woefully out of touch with recent developments and research into the efficacy of certain obstetric practices.

Health Visitors

A health visitor is a nurse who may also have midwifery qualifications, and who has in addition taken a special course in health visiting which includes counselling, sociology and child care and development. She is responsible for your care from around 10 days after the birth. Health visitors can also advise you about local support and specialist help if, for instance, you are feeling depressed or are having difficulty with breastfeeding.

Theoretically health visitors are the most accessible health professionals in the community, but many are grossly overworked. Although they are governed by the same body as midwives (the UKCC – United Kingdom Central Council for Nursing, Midwifery and Health Visiting), at present they are not required to keep their training up to date in the same way as midwives. Their system for ensuring continuing education is due to be over-hauled within the next five years. A good health visitor will be full of useful information, particularly about local mother-and-baby groups, activities and clinics, but unfortunately some are just as full of outdated or simply wrong advice. It's a matter of great concern that even a well-meaning health visitor can undermine breastfeeding with bad advice and give seriously unhelpful and rigid advice about your child's development.

Because health visitors are primarily there to identify households in the community where need is greatest – where there is a low income, a lack of education about basic good health, or where mother and/or baby is at risk from domestic violence or drug abuse – the questions which they ask can often seem threatening. The health visitor may feel as if she's just doing her job, but part of her job is also to use the evidence of her senses instead of a list of pre-set questions. Sadly, it's sometimes easier to ask inappropriate questions of healthy women than it is to intervene and support women who are obviously at risk or in need and whose social situation seems almost impossible to change.

Some mothers welcome a visit from the health visitor, but for others it can be something to dread. Some complain that their health visitor simply descended upon them out of the blue one day full of menacing questions about them and their baby. A health visitor should not simply drop in on you – though in practice many do. She should, if at all possible, make an appointment to see you at a mutually convenient time. You do not have to let her in if she does drop by. In fact, you are under no obligation to see her at all if you don't want to. If you want to avoid these ad hoc visits you can write to her at the clinic, ask her not to call on you and advise her that you will contact her if you need her. You don't have to attend any local clinics or groups which she may direct you to.

Advantages:

* Being visited by a health visitor can make a woman feel as if she still has some contact, if not with the person than at least with the system within which she had her baby.

* HVs can be a mine of useful information about the local community, and some are genuinely sensitive and knowledgeable about issues such as breastfeeding, depression and child development.

Meeting the 'Experts'

Disadvantages:

* The disadvantages lie as much within the system of health visiting as they do with individuals, i.e. too few individuals pursuing too many problems.

* The fact that Health Visitors come from a nursing background has implications for the way they respond to mothers' problems. They have been trained to *act* when many mothers simply want them to *listen*.

* Health visitors are not required to keep their training up to date. So if you approach your health visitor with a problem (for instance with breastfeeding) there is a chance you'll get some bad advice.

* Health visitors are trained to look for things which are wrong or outside the norm – medically, emotionally, developmentally – as a result many will speak to you and ask questions from a very negative point of view. It's known as the 'When did you stop beating your child?' syndrome.

Paediatricians

A paediatrician is an expert in child health and development. There are different kinds of paediatricians, combining other disciplines, such as paediatric surgeons, paediatric psychologists, paediatric oncologists. You may never see or need to see one, though there is always a paediatrician on standby during those labours where the baby is deemed to be in distress, in multiple births (in higher-order multiple births there is often one paediatrician for each baby) or where the outcome as regards the health of the baby is in some doubt. You have the right to request a referral to a consultant paediatrician or a paediatric surgeon during your pregnancy if there is any doubt about the health of your baby after birth.

Babies are not like adults. They do not respond to disease or medication in the same way, they do not follow the same patterns of wellness or illness which adults do. They are subject to certain illnesses which are rare in adults. For all these reasons it may be reassuring to know you have access to a paediatrician or a GP with extensive paediatric training or experience once the baby is born.

There are a proliferation of 'well-baby' and 'mother-and-baby' clinics all around the country staffed by health visitors and GPs. Any doctor can set up one of these clinics even if he has no real training or continuing educational qualifications in paediatrics. The same rule applies for paediatricians as for general practitioners: check what his qualifications are before letting him loose on your child.

Unfortunately in the UK, unlike Australia and the US, general practitioners cannot take a diploma in paediatrics. When a general practitioner trains, a component in paediatrics, or child surveillance, will have been compulsory, but this training could have taken place so many years ago that your doctor's knowledge may be terribly out of date. Equally your GP might be relatively young, newly out of medical school, and much of his knowledge will have been acquired from books rather than from actually having to deal with the problems of children and their effects on parents. Before allowing him to treat your child, ask what your GP does to keep his training up to date so that you can make an informed decision about whether you want your child to be seen by him. If you are not satisfied with the answer there is nothing to prevent you from registering your child with a different doctor from the rest of the family if you feel that it would be of benefit for your child to be seen by someone with more up-to-date knowledge about child health.

Advantages:

✳ Paediatricians are experts in child health and can reassure you that all is well and act swiftly if your child is ill.

Meeting the 'Experts'

* A doctor with paediatric experience is much more likely to be supportive of breastfeeding.

* A paediatrician is the best person to consult when your child is seriously ill. He or she can diagnose and refer you on to other specialist treatment as needed.

* A really good paediatrician, or doctor with paediatric experience, will not automatically prescribe antibiotics, antihistamines or pain-killers at the first sign of illness. All these things are often provided more for the relief of the parents (or doctors) than for the child, in whom they can occasionally produce serious side-effects.

Disadvantages:

* Paediatricians, like obstetricians, can suffer from only ever seeing children when they are ill. They may tend to prescribe treatments and medications too freely, when what may be more appropriate is consistent parental support while an illness runs its course.

* If you elect to book your child under another GP in your local area, your own GP may feel this is a slight upon his professional credentials and strike you and the rest of your family off his register.

Students

During the course of her pregnancy a woman will come into contact with medical and/or midwifery students. You have the right to refuse to have a consultation with a student. Likewise you can refuse to allow a student to perform any procedure on you. No student should undertake a diagnosis or procedure on you without a senior member of staff present. It is highly likely that when you go to a hospital for an appointment with the consultant you will be attended by an SHO, a student with a fancy title doing his or her residency on the obstetrics ward! If you are not sure whom you are having a consultation with – ask.

It is, of course, true that students learn by experience, but if you have strong misgivings about being a guinea pig, speak up. Equally you may feel that you would like to help in the training of students. If you feel that a student might benefit from participating in your labour you can agree to one being present. Some women who feel very strongly about having a natural birth, or giving birth in a different way, such as in water, are equally committed to helping both established and training practitioners to gain experience in attending these types of birth. Under such circumstances it may be best to ask that the student is present for the whole of your labour so that he or she may gain an understanding of the course of a normal labour.

In line with the recommendations in the Patient's Charter regarding informed consent, some teaching hospitals put up notices for mothers about their policies for student training. While most of these seem friendly enough on first reading, closer scrutiny often reveals a degree of coercion. Usually they emphasize the importance of a woman's co-operation in order to train future members of the health profession. They may innocently state that they know you 'won't mind' if a student is present during an ante-natal visit, because it forms such a 'valuable' part of his or her training.

In order truly to inform women of their rights, and thus enable them to make an informed decision about student participation in their ante-natal care or labour, any such notice should say something along the lines of:

> This hospital provides training for medical and midwifery students. During your visits and stay here you may be approached for permission for them to attend a consultation or to be involved in your care, e.g. delivering your baby under supervision. You may agree or refuse. The decision is entirely yours and your future care will in no way be

affected by that decision. If you wish you may ask for your decision to be recorded in your case notes.[12]

Booking into a teaching hospital does not imply that you have given your automatic consent to being attended by medical or midwifery students – although far too many doctors think it does. Neither can you be required to sign away your right to say 'no'. Your consent must be sought and given before any student becomes involved in your care.

Advantages:

✳ Student training is part of the larger, professional continuum of the birth process. No one can tell in advance what a birth will be like, but if you are planning to have the kind of birth which might enhance a student's understanding of the process – at home, in water, a vaginal breech – you may like to invite him or her to attend you or be present during your labour.

✳ Many students, particularly midwifery students, still have an element of enthusiasm about birth. It can be a pleasure to be around this kind of person.

Disadvantages:

✳ It is an unfortunate fact of training in a hospital setting that medical and midwifery students hardly ever get to see normal, physiological births. They repeatedly get trotted in to observe 'interesting' cases (twins, breeches, retained placentas, haemorrhaging women, etc.) instead and can end up feeling frustrated by their inability to get involved and fearful of what is being presented to them as the unpredictability of the birth process.

Every Woman's BirthRights

* Students performing delicate procedures such as cutting or stitching up a perineum are not always given the best supervision. This can result in real and lasting damage to a woman's body.

* Some routine procedures (episiotomies, amniotomies, vaginal examinations, etc.) are performed more for the benefit of students than for the good of the mother or her baby.

* If you are not very clear about what you will and will not allow vis-à-vis students, you may find that the consultant will march in on you, without knocking, in the middle of your labour, with half a dozen students in tow and begin lecturing them. This can be very upsetting. You are not an 'interesting case', you are a person and you have the right to throw all of them (including the consultant) out.

Good Practitioners and Good Patients

Old habits die hard, and although the maternity services are improving and attitudes are changing, mothers, doctors and midwives are all, to some extent, locked into perceived roles which are hard to break out of. This is why when a woman finds the strength to break out of her role as a passive recipient of care she can meet with such disapproval from those around her.

The traits that define a 'good' practitioner, for many women, are personality and social skills rather than professional ability.[13] This may in part be due to the fact that many women don't feel able, or don't feel they have a right to, for instance, make a judgement about a doctor's clinical skills. But it is important to remember that the standards which might apply to other areas of medical care are often inappropriate in the realm of maternity care. If a woman doesn't feel able to judge clinicians' skills or question their actions, it is usually only because a lack of self-confidence, resulting from the dearth of relevant information about rights and choices and what is and is not 'normal', prohibits her from speaking out.

This fear can prevent women from asking for a second opinion – something which every woman has a right to. Fear can stop women from refusing procedures which they are uncomfortable with, or from insisting that a test result which they feel might be wrong is confirmed by a different practitioner using different equipment. It can prevent them from finding a new practitioner, even if the care they are currently receiving is unacceptable.

For the most part women's fears about speaking up for themselves and being decisive often centre around things like 'bothering the busy doctors with little things'; 'hurting the doctor's feelings' by rejecting his advice; being seen as 'difficult' or 'uncooperative'; being less educated than the doctor; not knowing the 'language'; being made to look foolish by his 'logical' arguments; losing the argument; no immediate reward for being assertive; and fear of shouldering the often overwhelming responsibility for their unborn baby's health and well-being.

Mothers' reluctance to be more assertive can also centre around a feeling of guilt or a misplaced sense of responsibility for the feelings of others. Without intending to, many women end up caring for their carers. Women, who are so used to listening to and helping to solve other people's problems, can easily be manipulated into taking responsibility for their practitioners. Women have told me stories of midwives talking over them in labour: 'Oh I'm so tired, this labour has gone on far too long. I'll never be able to take my clinic tomorrow. Let me help you speed it up a bit' or doctors making appeals to them: 'The last woman who came in here wanting a water birth ended up with a post-partum haemorrhage. I can't tell you how upset I was. You wouldn't want to put me through that again, would you?' This puts the mother in the impossible position of having to 'rescue' the practitioner. A woman caught in the midst of the internal conflicts and guilt which can arise as she tries to please both herself and her practitioner, can be more easily influenced and manipulated into doing what the practitioner thinks is right instead of what she thinks is right.

It cannot be said often enough: when it comes to pregnancy and childbirth, women know best what's right for them and what's not. Yet often women shrink from speaking up or criticizing their doctors. When a doctor is rude or offhand, if he does not listen or makes a mistake, we are much more likely to excuse his behaviour by saying, 'Well, he's a busy man' or 'It must be hard having to see all those people every day.' When a doctor seems kind there is a tendency to put it down to luck or to catching him on a good day. Comments like 'He's very tolerant' or 'I hated to bother him with it really', as if the doctor is some sort of imposing father figure, are not uncommon. The same assumptions apply to midwives, who sometimes become mother figures who are 'only doing what's best for you, dear'. Both scenarios place women in an inferior position which can be difficult to break out of.

Not surprisingly, some doctors and midwives also have their own ideas about what a good patient is. All too often, and perhaps inevitably given the sexual and power politics which are so much a part of the system, she is passive. Quite often she is an uneducated, 'working-class' woman who lays no claim to special knowledge. One way or another, she accepts that the doctor or midwife knows best, and does what she is told. She 'just gets on with the job without any airy-fairy notions of fulfilment and satisfaction, recognizing that it is the end product that matters rather than the process'.[14]

In addition to the stereotype of the good patient, pregnant women have to work against another set of beliefs which prevents them from being taken seriously: that pregnant women are emotionally unstable, that they are incapable of rational thought, that they are weak and inconsistent and, especially if it is their first baby, naïve.[15]

In a busy labour ward, stereotypes can replace the time-consuming process of getting to know individuals. Because medical education places so little value on communication skills, stereotype becomes the main frame of reference for many practitioners. It is the tool they use to help them deal with the

Meeting the 'Experts'

continual influx of different personality types from a variety of social and ethnic backgrounds who come through their doors every day. So, a woman who is educated and assertive becomes 'one of those NCT types'; a woman who wants an active birth probably wants to have her baby 'squatting in a field' or 'hanging from the chandelier'; mothers from some ethnic groups are characterized as 'complaining' or 'lazy', and so it goes.

The first person to look at when considering who will care for you throughout your pregnancy and birth is you. Determine what you want your own role to be in your and your baby's care. Do you want to be involved and have some measure of control and a say in what is done to you? Or would you feel more secure turning over some or all of your care to someone else?

You may also want to examine your own stereotypes of what a good doctor or a good midwife is. Are you looking for your healthcare practitioners to fulfil a role which could be more readily fulfilled by a friend, a partner, a parent or even yourself? Pay attention to the ways in which you traditionally react to authority figures. Do you look them straight in the eye or do you avert your gaze, lower your voice, placate them – in fact do whatever it takes to get through the examination quickly and without a fuss? Are you comfortable with the your ante-natal care and labour being a reflection of this, or would you like a change? Your needs and views will determine what kind of practitioner will serve your needs best during pregnancy and birth.

3
The Ante-natal Routine

Ante-natal care is a 20th-century invention. It was initially established in the hope of finding those women whose labours might become complicated by conditions which arose and, in some cases, could be helped during pregnancy. As science and technology evolved, ante-natal care expanded to include diagnostic tests to detect fetal abnormalities. Education about the consequences of certain infectious diseases such as Rubella, venereal disease and urinary tract infections, and how to avoid them, was also seen as important. The expected result of this intensive care programme was that it would reduce maternal and neonatal deaths and the incidence of abnormalities through either corrective action during pregnancy or by aborting a fetus before it reached full-term.

In addition, ante-natal care was seen as a way of introducing women, particularly those who were generally uneducated and living in poorer circumstances, to the principles of good health during pregnancy. Of course, the principles of good health in pregnancy do not differ from those at any other time in a woman's life. Adequate nutrition, good personal hygiene, moderate exercise, periods of activity, rest and sleep as well as freedom from excessive amounts of stress are all it takes, in most cases, to ensure the health of both mother and baby. Unfortunately, these prerequisites are far more easily met by women in higher socio-economic groups, who have the necessary economic, educational and practical resources. Women in less fortunate circumstances, the ones whom ante-natal care is supposed to support, struggle even today to attain them.

More recently, with the discovery of concepts such as continuity of care and carer, the ante-natal period is also perceived as a time when a mother can get to know her doctor or midwife and form a reasonable relationship with him or her.

So What Are They Looking For?

Women experience two different types of difficulties during pregnancy: those which are transient and are unlikely to result in serious complications (and which may, if looked at in a different light, be seen as normal physiological reactions to pregnancy), and those which could, if left unchecked, end up complicating labour and possibly even result in damage or death to either mother or baby.

The transient symptoms of pregnancy are well documented. They include nausea, vomiting, sweating, muscle cramps, vertigo, headaches, frequent urination, constipation, tingling hands and legs, varicose veins, bleeding gums, sinusitis, insomnia, water retention and more. The frequency of these symptoms and the fact that they are not life-threatening has meant that they are seen as a normal part of pregnancy; as such, medical researchers have done little to find out who suffers the most from what and why.

Potentially more serious conditions include placenta praevia, malpresentation of the baby, true pelvic or fetal head disproportion, pre-eclampsia, growth retardation and fetal abnormalities. In addition, multiple pregnancy and certain aspects of the mother's lifestyle – whether or not she smokes, drinks, takes drugs or has a poor diet – can contribute to potential problems. What distinguishes these from the transient symptoms of pregnancy is that, if not properly managed and under certain circumstances, they can result in damage to both mother and baby. It is this damage that ante-natal surveillance is supposed to prevent.

The detection of anomalies in the mother's health during pregnancy certainly has a place in modern ante-natal care. Early diagnosis and management of conditions such as pre-eclampsia – which can develop into eclampsia, a potentially lethal condition peculiar to pregnancy – has meant many more mothers have lived to see their babies born. The detection of babies in difficult positions and the existence of two or more babies in the womb (multiple pregnancy) has meant that doctors and midwives, in theory at least, can respond to and manage individual cases more appropriately.

There is also an assumption that early detection of fetal abnormalities gives women greater freedom to choose, for instance, whether they will keep or abort a baby with certain types of abnormalities (although many severely abnormal fetuses will spontaneously abort before 20 weeks anyway). For the woman who chooses to keep her baby there is more time to adjust to how the baby will be. For the woman who does not, it is assumed that early abortion has fewer emotional and physiological consequences, though obviously the emotional impact of a termination varies between individuals.

Whether the ante-natal routine actually helps prevent maternal and neonatal deaths or abnormalities is not something about which there is any conclusive proof. Maternal and perinatal mortality in Britain first began to go down during the Second World War when, ironically, there was an acute shortage of doctors and personal stress and anxiety must have created complications in pregnancy and labour, but the national diet was much healthier. In addition, fresh milk and vitamin supplements for pregnant and nursing mothers were subsidized, and extra amounts of rationed foods like eggs were made available to these women. This, it could be argued, made the biggest difference to the overall health of mothers and babies.

One thing constant medical attention does do effectively, however, is to convince pregnant women that death and danger are just around the corner. Women who have to go frequently to a hospital or clinic for tests are not in the same shape, emotionally or psychologically, as those who do not. Not surprisingly, this notion that something could go wrong at any minute has never been borne out by research. For instance, in reviewing perinatal death statistics since 1958, Marjorie Tew has observed that, in spite of increased ante-natal vigilance, figures for intrauterine growth retardation have hardly changed.[1] In 1958, 6.7 per cent of babies weighing under 2,500 g ($5^{1}/_{2}$ lb) accounted for 53 per cent of all perinatal deaths. In 1990, 6.8 per cent of these low-birthweight babies made up 59.3 per cent of all perinatal deaths!

Stress is a major contributing factor to problems in pregnancy. Yet we seldom acknowledge the fact that women who are being continuously screened ante-natally can feel they are under a great deal of stress. This, in turn, can contribute to problems such as pre-eclampsia, depression and anaemia. Women under stress may drink, smoke or eat more, and these things will affect the course of pregnancy. In addition, the environment in which ante-natal care is conducted can do little to put mothers at ease. Ante-natal clinics have always been the same. The idea that the overcrowding, lack of comfort, long waiting times, hurried visits and inadequate explanations which many women experience today are indicative of the busy modern world we live in, is simply not true. Hospitals and clinics have never been organized to receive the number of pregnant women who come through their doors each year. A Government Board memorandum circulated in 1915 suggests that 'Crowding, and protracted waiting of mothers and their children, should be avoided, and the interview of the doctor with each mother and child should not be hurried.'[2]

In 1949 things were not much better. As one mother wrote of her ante-natal experience:

> The corridor is very long, patterned by a bewildering array of doors. Mothers, hastily directed, are forever losing

The Ante-natal Routine

themselves through these apertures: going through the third door on the left instead of the second door on the right, like cows bewildered by a strange byre. Whenever this happens a nurse ... bursts out of nowhere and tweaks the unfortunate back with loud but cheerful cries of: 'Not there, dear, not there! But *there*.'[3]

Again, in 1961, it was determined that:

The commonest cause of dissatisfaction during the ante-natal period seems to be the long waiting times, often hours spent in poor, overcrowded premises, followed by a rapid examination with no real privacy. Another frequent complaint is either the lack of explanation of abnormalities which have arisen ... or a partial explanation which gives rise to worry.[4]

Most women sitting in ante-natal clinics today will recognize that little has changed. But apart from being exasperating, the environment in which ante-natal care is given can also give rise to the problems of over-diagnosis and under-diagnosis, both of which can disadvantage mothers and babies. Looking for problems in pregnancy can become a self-fulfilling prophecy. It may be that in order to justify the time and the money we spend looking for problems, we make sure we find them. Practitioners who see pregnancy as pathological rather than physiological may misinterpret test results and diagnose problems where there are none, or apply interventions where symptoms are transient and self-correcting. These interventions sometimes bring their own risks (see Chapter 4) and occasionally, when their debilitating side-effects compromise the health of the mother or baby, a practitioner may even add insult to injury by saying, 'I told you so.'

The other side of this is the busy ante-natal clinic where the majority of women are healthy and well. Practitioners under these circumstances can be lulled into complacency, missing obvious problems and mismanaging women who genuinely need help.

Caught up in the ante-natal routine, it can be easy to lose sight of the fact that care only benefits women if it is appropriate. We also tend to miss the obvious truth that the way women care for themselves, and the way they are cared for by their family and friends, may in the end have a greater impact on their continued health, and that of their babies, than almost anything medicine can offer.

The Baby's Well-being

There are now a whole range of tests to assess a baby's well-being. Initially this might seem very reassuring. But the truth is that, while doctors can diagnose certain abnormalities, there is very little they can do to correct them, short of offering the mother a termination.

When a mother can feel her baby moving inside her it is both exciting and terrifying. Exciting because the child seems more 'real' to her, but terrifying because fears that the child may be deformed or abnormal in some way may also become more real. Her fears may be exacerbated by unthinking (and insensitive) professionals who, in their dogged search for the abnormal, make off-hand comments like, 'The baby's quite small, dear,' 'I can't find the heartbeat. Have you felt the baby move lately?' Often these comments are made and then dismissed as being unimportant. If a practitioner makes a comment like this to you, you have a right to a full explanation. If he can't provide one, you can remind him that he should be more thoughtful in what he says to you.

Abnormalities

The first thing which many mothers say when their child is born, regardless of how healthy they are, how uncomplicated their pregnancy was and how healthy the baby seemed *in utero*, is 'Is he/she all right?' The vast majority of babies are, of course, 'all right'. Recent figures show that the actual number of babies born with congenital malformations is 91.4 per 10,000 births.[5]

The Ante-natal Routine

The occurrence of major abnormalities is:

Central nervous system malformations	4.7 per 10,000
Anencephaly	0.5 per 10,000
Spina Bifida	1.2 per 10,000
Hydrocephalus	1.5 per 10,000
Cleft lip and/or palate	7.1 per 10,000
Cleft palate only	3.5 per 10,000
Cardiovascular malformations	7.7 per 10,000
Hydrospadies and epispadies	8.0 per 10,000
Club Foot	11.0 per 10,000
Down's Syndrome	5.7 per 10,000

Obviously these figures say nothing about the degrees to which babies might be affected. Some handicaps are not life-threatening and can be corrected *in utero* or shortly after birth. Equally, they do not take into account those babies who were either diagnosed as abnormal and medically terminated, or those which were spontaneously aborted. Even so, for the majority of mothers the chance of having a handicapped or otherwise abnormal baby is very small. But, as Sheila Kitzinger puts it:

> Almost every expectant mother has also wondered at some time, perhaps in the dead of night, when she is most alone, how she would react to her baby being born dead and whether she could face it. For some pregnant women it is a nagging fear which holds threat of punishment for negative

feelings that they have had about the baby and becoming a mother. Perhaps the baby was conceived before it was really convenient, and the woman thought of having a termination and now feels guilty that she even considered it. Perhaps she was pregnant before, and that pregnancy was terminated, maybe for good reasons, but the abortion casts its shadow forward onto the present pregnancy ... There must be few women who have not thought occasionally that pregnancy was a nuisance or been apprehensive at the thought of having to cope with a baby and the drastic change in life-style necessitated by its arrival. Women punish themselves for feelings of rejection with fantasies of the child being born dead or being physically or mentally handicapped.[6]

A woman's attitude to and experience of disability may greatly influence her perception of the risk of producing a handicapped child. A woman who has been exposed to children with physical or mental disabilities, either through work, family or friends, may feel more 'at risk' even if there is no 'logical' reason to. A woman who has no such experience may not have the same fears.

For a mother who does end up giving birth to a child with abnormalities, the figures may provide not so much reassurance as statistical punishment. She may feel singled out and wonder why, if so few babies are born handicapped, hers had to be one of them? She may feel cheated by the very system of care which so confidently boasted that it could accurately diagnose abnormalities with an increasing battery of tests.

Everyone has his or her own opinions on the subject of abnormalities, and it can sometimes be difficult to get all the facts. There are, however, many groups, such as Support after Termination for Foetal Abnormality (SAFTA) and Kith and Kids, which a woman can turn to for support and information.

Fetal Size and Fetal Growth
The baby's size at any point during your pregnancy is used primarily to determine its age and its rate of growth – though size

The Ante-natal Routine

and growth are not the same thing. It's important to make the distinction between those babies who are growing but consistently fall below the accepted norm for size, known as 'light for dates' babies, and those who do not gain weight or whose weight falls suddenly below the norm within a short period of time and are therefore potentially affected by intrauterine growth retardation.

Assessing fetal growth is not an exact science. While there is evidence that the majority of babies follow a predictable growth curve during the first three months of pregnancy, after then individual babies tend to follow their own course, punctuated by unpredictable periods of stasis and growth. Growth charts (which it is assumed all babies have read and will conform to) do not take into account the relative size of the parents, inherited or genetic factors such as ethnic group, or the lifestyle of the mother.

Nevertheless, doctors feel that monitoring the baby's size is important. Certainly small babies are more likely to die than large ones. One in 15 babies is born weighing under 2,500 g (5^{1}/$_{2}$lb), and these babies account for 60 per cent of neonatal deaths.[7] But there are a number of factors which may influence these figures. Doctors who have diagnosed growth retardation are often too quick to induce labour. Early induction means that these babies are not only small for dates, but may be born prematurely and less able to cope with life outside the womb. Since there is no cure for intrauterine growth retardation, the practice of early induction or elective delivery seems to be questionable. There is no evidence that substituting a special care baby unit for a womb does any good in these circumstances.[8]

Initially, ultrasound scans are used to assess the baby's age and establish an estimated delivery date (EDD). As time goes on, practitioners may use repeated scans to detect signs of possible growth retardation and, less importantly, to predict the baby's eventual birthweight. Predicting a baby's birthweight is in fact almost impossible and a pointless exercise. It is also an entirely different issue from detecting a growth-retarded baby. It also appears that repeated scanning for small babies may create the very problem it sets out to solve.

One large, randomized controlled trial, the purpose of which was to demonstrate the safety of repeated scanning, found some disturbing results. In a group of 2,834 women, 1,415 were scanned with ultrasound and Doppler at 18, 24, 28, 34 and 38 weeks, while the other 1,419 were given a single ultrasound scan at 18 weeks. The only difference between the two groups was a 30 per cent higher rate of intrauterine growth retardation in the *scanned* group. The authors concluded that: 'It would seem prudent to limit ultrasound examinations of the fetus to those cases in which the information is likely to be of clinical value.'[9]

Growth-retarded babies may move less, which is the rationale behind kick charts. But kick charts, as a preventative measure, are not very useful. Fetal death *may* occur swiftly, a day or so after the baby stops moving. But it is also likely that the baby may never stop moving and simply die. Reduced movement may be the baby's way of conserving precious energy. During this time blood flow is redistributed away from the liver and kidneys to the brain and heart. This is why using ultrasound to measure the diameter of the baby's head in suspected cases of growth retardation may give misleading results, since the brain is the organ whose growth is often the least affected by the condition.

Intrauterine growth retardation is likely to be caused by a number of factors. Chief among these is a decrease in the quantity and quality of nourishment which the baby is receiving via the placenta. It is known that some mothers are more at risk than others. Those who smoke, drink, who habitually use drugs and who, for whatever reason, have a poor diet, and those who are subject to high amounts of stress, have a greater chance of having a growth-retarded baby. Many congenitally malformed babies are also growth retarded.

When it comes to large babies of 4,000 g (8 lb 13 oz) or more, doctors look for the possibility of diabetes. However, if there is no family history of the disease and the mother does not have diabetes or some form of pregnancy-induced glucose intolerance, this is unlikely. Even in mothers who do have diabetes, there is only a small chance of it being passed on to the baby.

The Ante-natal Routine

Some babies are simply big. The real reason why doctors are so concerned about big babies is that they are afraid of complications during delivery such as shoulder dystocia (when the baby's head is born and the body then becomes stuck at the shoulders). However, the size of the baby is not a good indication of the risk of shoulder dystocia. Half of the cases of shoulder dystocia are to babies weighing less than 4,000 g (8 lb 13 oz).[10]

The usual consequence for a woman whose baby is stuck at the shoulders is to put her in the lithotomy position (on her back with her legs well supported) and perform a large episiotomy, or to push the baby back up inside her and deliver it by caesarean. This can result in unusually high levels of injury and illness for both mother and baby. In the US, midwives have found that putting the mother on all fours for this type of complication generally results in an easy delivery, with little or no injury to mother or baby.[11]

Twins and Multiple Pregnancies

Twins are not necessarily a medical emergency, though they are often treated as such. Multiple pregnancies, especially if they are the result of an IVF programme, may provide more legitimate reasons to worry. While the tabloids celebrate these miracles of modern medicine, the dark, often unreported truth is that many of these babies do not arrive in this world in very good shape. They often have mental and physical handicaps as well as learning disabilities. The financial and emotional impact of multiple pregnancies on parents is illustrated by the fact that so many of these babies end up in foster homes.

Multiple pregnancies are more prone to medical problems such as poor fetal growth (though these babies are naturally smaller than others), the risk of preterm delivery, and premature death. In addition, one or more of the babies may be in a difficult position. These possibilities lead many practitioners to recommend caesarean delivery as a matter of routine, though there is no hard evidence to show that this is always the best course for either mother or babies. For the mother, the unpleasant physical symptoms of pregnancy are usually experienced to a greater degree. Emotionally and psychologically she may also be more anxious which, in turn, may lead to more problems during pregnancy.

Mothers of twins are often advised to rest. There is little evidence to show that this has much of a beneficial effect on outcomes, in fact there is some evidence that it can increase the risk of spontaneous preterm labour and low birthweight, possibly because long periods of bed rest can compromise blood flow to the placenta. What is true is that mothers with two or more babies need a great deal more emotional and practical support during pregnancy, birth and postnatally. Should the mother of twins choose to have a vaginal birth, home birth or water labour and birth, for instance (and there is no real reason why, if she and her babies are well, she should not), she will have twice the fight on her hands to achieve it.

For a mother of twins or more the biggest emergency may be, in the end, an emotional one, even if she is happy with the idea. Mothers who are diagnosed as having twins or more often feel a sense of shock and will need time to adjust all their expectations of birth and of life afterwards. Organizations such as the Twins and Multiple Births Association (TAMBA) and the NCT can help with practical advice and by putting mothers in touch with other women in a similar situation.

Fetal Position

Babies twist and turn into all kinds of positions in the womb throughout pregnancy. Towards the end of pregnancy the majority of babies settle head down with their backs facing towards the left of their mother's abdomen (this is known as the left occipito anterior position). While this is the most common, it is not the only normal position. Most of the other positions which babies can take up do not necessarily present any danger to them or their mothers and do not usually require any medical intervention, although a baby whose back is facing its mother's back during labour can cause a painful type of labour called backache

The Ante-natal Routine

labour, for which an epidural during the early part of labour *may* prove helpful for some.

The two positions which send practitioners into surgical overdrive, however, are the breech presentation (bottom or feet first) and the transverse presentation (lying horizontally). While the latter may be an indication that a caesarean is necessary, the former rarely is.

Between 29 and 32 weeks, approximately 15 per cent of babies are in the breech position. Only 3 to 4 per cent of these persist into labour. As your pregnancy progresses there is less and less chance that a breech will turn into a head-down (or cephalic) position spontaneously.

Because it has become the norm to perform a caesarean for babies in a breech position, many midwives have become deskilled in delivering these babies vaginally. When a practitioner says that a vaginal delivery of a breech baby is unsafe, that your pelvis is too small or your baby is too big, what he or she may really be saying is 'I don't know how to do it.' The only way to tell if you can deliver your baby vaginally is by a trial of labour. If the first stage progresses well, then there is no reason why you should not go on to deliver vaginally without risk to you or your baby. A breech baby does not contraindicate birth at home, though it would be wise to make sure that you have a midwife who is experienced in this type of delivery.

If your doctor doesn't immediately recommend an elective caesarean for a breech baby, he may recommend an *external version* – an attempt to turn the baby by applying gentle pressure on the mother's abdomen. On the whole these are more successful when performed in labour rather than late in pregnancy. Few practitioners will actually try and turn a baby in labour, though, because they generally like to perform a version with the aid of a muscle relaxant and this, of course, is contraindicated in labour. However, if the mother is relaxed and the practitioner is skilled (and the latter is a big IF), it is not necessary to use drugs. Before term there is thought to be a 1 per cent chance that the baby could die during the procedure. In labour this is greatly reduced and there is a 75 per cent chance that the mother will go on to deliver vaginally. Versions performed on a woman who has gone into labour spontaneously have been shown to reduce the caesarean rates for breeches considerably. One study showed that, at the most conservative estimate, external version performed on all breech babies in labour would prevent 34 per cent of all breech deliveries and 14 per cent of all caesareans for breech.[12]

Many practitioners have lost the skill of turning breech babies. If you want a doctor to try and turn your baby, find one who is experienced. In unskilled hands there is a chance of detaching the placenta during the procedure. Your practitioners should use ultrasound to check your baby's (and your placenta's) position. Some babies revert to their breech position after an apparently successful version, so you will need to weigh up the pros and cons of an attempted version carefully.

Most doctors will not 'allow' a woman with a breech baby to go into labour spontaneously. They argue that there is a risk to the baby because its head will not have the time to mould itself slowly to the shape of the mother's pelvis, possibly causing trauma and/or brain damage. Some doctors brow-beat mothers with the terrifying picture of the baby's body hanging from her vagina, its head stuck in her pelvis. The chance of this happening is so rare that there are not even any figures to show how often it occurs. The final decision for delivering your breech baby is *yours*, not your doctors. Generally speaking, if the baby's body delivers easily then there should be no problem delivering the head. In cases like this, obstetric management of labour, with the woman on her back or propped up on a delivery bed, is a great disadvantage. The mother will need to 'open up' her pelvis and this can only be done if she is in a full or supported squat. Not only do you have the right to a trial of labour with a breech baby, you have a reasonable chance of success. If your practitioner refuses, ask to be referred to the care of someone who has a more sympathetic point of view.

When your baby is a breech it may be wise to take more care than usual to assess what your own individual risk is. This will

The Ante-natal Routine

entail getting all the information you can about the estimated size of the baby, its neck flexion (in other words, whether its chin is tucked neatly onto its chest or sticking out) and the *estimated* size of your pelvis. But in the end all of these things are mere guesswork. One survey, looking at the outcomes for both diagnosed breeches and undiagnosed breeches, found that those babies who were undiagnosed and delivered vaginally actually fared as well, and in some cases better, than those who had been diagnosed early and had all the 'benefit' of obstetric management.[13]

If your baby is diagnosed as being in a transverse lie, there is no need to panic about how your baby will be delivered before you go into labour. Less than 20 per cent of those babies diagnosed as being transverse before 32 weeks are still in this position at term. It is possible to turn the baby in labour, as you might for a breech baby, but there is less chance of success. Babies who persist in a transverse presentation will need to be delivered by caesarean section. Reasons for a baby turning into a transverse lie include multiple pregnancy, an abnormally small womb, fetal abnormality, a shortening of the length of the uterus because the placenta is sited either at the top or the bottom of the uterus, and anything which may prevent the baby settling into the pelvis, such as pelvic fibroids, tumours or cysts.

If your baby is in a breech or transverse position, you could try some self-help methods during pregnancy such as the knee-chest position (on all fours resting your head on the floor, with your bottom in the air), lots of vigorous walking, acupuncture, or acupressure. Sometimes these things work. But probably the most positive action you can take is just to accept it and, if your baby is in a breech position, start collecting all the information you can about breech deliveries. More and more observers are beginning to accept the idea that babies who persist in difficult positions have made a 'choice' to be born in a different way. However primitive and unfathomable this primal process may be, we should respect it and not try to control or correct it with invasive procedures such as the external version. Our children don't always do what we want them to – parents of breech and transverse lie babies learn this earlier than most.

The Mother's Well-being

Concern for the mother's well-being is often just a veiled concern for the baby. This is why it is sometimes experienced as being very clinical and impersonal. It is often another way of making sure that the 'container' is in optimum shape to deliver healthy 'contents'. The main things which your practitioner will be looking for are pre-eclampsia, anaemia, glucose intolerance, and placenta praevia. Most of these are, thankfully, rare, and in most cases do not pose a great threat to either mother or baby if monitored carefully.

Pre-eclampsia

Even though it only affects between 5 and 10 per cent of pregnant women, every ante-natal test is geared up to search and search again for this condition, which is unique to pregnancy. Yet few women actually know what it is or how it might affect them or their babies. What's more, few experts actually have a much better understanding of it.

Pre-eclampsia is and has been known by a number of different names all over the world. It can be referred to as pre-eclamptic toxaemia or PET, as pregnancy-induced hypertension or PIH, toxaemia, hypertensive disease of pregnancy or HDP, metabolic toxaemia of late pregnancy or MTLP, and even gestosis. The overabundance of names should be enough to indicate a certain amount of confusion about what exactly it is and how it develops.

The first indication which practitioners look for is hypertension (raised blood pressure). Should a woman also have oedema (swelling due to water retention) and raised levels of uric acid in the blood, there is cause for concern. Together these symptoms generally indicate pre-eclampsia, singly they do not usually pose a threat.

The Ante-natal Routine

If early symptoms of pre-eclampsia are left untreated, protein may eventually appear in the urine. (Even diagnosing this can be a bit hit and miss. It is known that the dipsticks used to detect protein in a woman's urine have a 25 per cent false positive rate, when only traces of protein are indicated.[14]) When this happens, clots and fatty acids can build up in the placenta, interfering with its efficiency and eventually causing it to cease functioning altogether. When the placenta is not functioning properly the baby is not getting essential oxygen and nutrients, and growth retardation is a real possibility. Under these circumstances the body may, as a survival mechanism, instigate labour prematurely. Nearly 30 per cent of cases of pre-eclampsia are first detected in labour, either because they were missed by ante-natal screening or because the condition did not manifest until then.

True pre-eclampsia can be dangerous and if left untreated can develop into full-blown eclampsia – a potentially lethal condition for both mother and baby. This is rare – about 1 in 2,000 cases of pre-eclampsia turn into eclampsia. Early symptoms include severe headaches, flashing lights, nausea, vomiting and pain in the abdomen. In very extreme cases the mother may experience fits, convulsions and, more rarely, go into a coma. If you experience any of the symptoms of eclampsia, get yourself to your midwife or doctor immediately and have your blood and urine tested. Don't be put off by anyone who tells you these are normal symptoms of pregnancy – they aren't. Demand that the proper tests are carried out, without delay. If for any reason your doctor or midwife refuses, get yourself to hospital.

What Causes Pre-eclampsia?

Considering how worried doctors are about women developing pre-eclampsia, it is surprising how little research there is about it. Pre-eclampsia is more common in first pregnancies and usually shows itself in middle to late pregnancy (except in women who have been malnourished for years). Women who have diabetes or kidney disease, high blood pressure, are carrying twins or more, those with a family history of high blood pressure or pre-eclampsia, women over 40, those who suffer from migraine and those who had pre-eclampsia in a previous pregnancy are most at risk. A woman's partner also seems to have some influence on this condition. Provided she is with the same partner, her chances of developing pre-eclampsia decline with each pregnancy. However, if a woman has her second or subsequent baby with a different man, the chances of developing pre-eclampsia are the same as if she were having her first baby.

Other theories include the idea that some placentas have narrower blood vessels than others, thus predisposing the mothers to the disease, that in some mothers the immune system views the baby as a foreign body and is trying to reject it, and that what we call pre-eclampsia is a normal physiological adaptation to pregnancy. But perhaps the single biggest factor which has been linked to pre-eclampsia is poor diet: it is more likely to develop in women who are very undernourished and living in a stressful environment.

Can It Be Cured?

In mild to moderate forms pre-eclampsia does not pose a particular threat to either mother or baby – particularly if carefully monitored. The usual advice is for the mother to have plenty of bed rest. If she finds it hard to do this at home (and few mothers can, especially since at this stage they will feel relatively fit and well) then she is usually asked to come into hospital. Unfortunately stress is a major contributing factor to pre-eclampsia. Many women find the stress and, if they are employed, the financial implications of being confined to bed, away from family and friends in hospital in the middle of their pregnancies more stressful than any self-imposed rest. There is not a shred of evidence to suggest that bed rest, however welcome it might be for some, is the answer to mild to moderate pre-eclampsia. We also need to consider the consequences of the stress and guilt which might result from telling an already over-burdened woman she should rest.

The Ante-natal Routine

Improved diet may be one way to prevent and halt the progress of pre-eclampsia.[15] Unfortunately, many practitioners are ignorant of what constitutes a proper diet for pregnancy. There has been very little research into how diet might prevent or improve pre-eclampsia, but since a poor diet is so often linked to its occurrence it would seem reasonable that an improved diet might make some difference – it certainly couldn't hurt! Taking good care of yourself is not an optional extra under these circumstances, it is a necessity. In desperation many women have turned to support organizations such as the Pre-eclamptic Toxaemia Society (PETS) for advice. This usually centres around advising the woman of her options and, if she is interested, providing details of a high-protein diet which has helped a number of women (known as the Brewer Diet, devised by American obstetrician, Dr Tom Brewer).

During your ante-natal care you may be advised to limit both your salt intake and weight gain in order to prevent pre-eclampsia. This is some of the most damaging advice there is. Pregnant women need salt as much as any of us. The greater volume of blood in a pregnant woman's body means that she will be sweating more and secreting more salt through her sweat. Salt helps regulate the fluid balance in the body and is essential for the proper functioning of nerves and muscles.

Pregnant women also need to follow the dictates of their appetites and gain as much weight as they need to gain. They also need to drink as much as they need to. Restricting fluid intake will not forestall the oedema which can be associated with pre-eclampsia. The majority of pregnant women, between 50–80 per cent, experience some form of water retention and swelling, usually in the ankles, feet, hands and face. Free intake of fluids can help keep your kidneys working well, flushing waste products out of your system. Most women who end up with pre-eclampsia live in circumstances where eating the proper food can be difficult and expensive. Ante-natal surveillance can identify them, but has not yet found a way of helping them. In contrast, there is absolutely no excuse for women who are relatively affluent to restrict their calorie intake in order to preserve their figures. There is plenty of evidence to show that restrictive dietary regimes, far from preventing pre-eclampsia, may actually end up causing it.

Doctors also use a number of drugs to combat pre-eclampsia and keep it from developing into full-blown eclampsia. With eclampsia there is debate among professionals as to what drug is best, with pre-eclampsia the debate is whether *any* drug is best. The kinds of drugs used include supplements of calcium and zinc, diuretics, low doses of aspirin, tranquillizers, mood-altering drugs, muscle relaxants (known as tocolytics, and used to forestall the onset of labour), drugs to reduce blood pressure (anti-hypertensive drugs) and drugs to thin the blood (anti-coagulants). There is very little evidence to show that any of these actually does much good.[16] The fewer drugs you take while you are pregnant, the better for you and your baby.

Tranquillizers and tocolytics can interfere with a mother's appetite, creating even more problems. Anti-hypertensive drugs can help to maintain a mother's blood pressure but cannot reduce it, nor can they prevent protein appearing in her urine, growth retardation, pre-term birth, or the likelihood of her having to have a caesarean section.

Does It Affect Labour?

Most doctors take what they feel is a very conservative approach to delivering the babies of mothers with pre-eclampsia. In other words, they like mothers to agree to an elective caesarean, preferably before term. Unless absolutely necessary a caesarean is an aggressive, not a conservative solution. Since pre-eclampsia is associated with growth retardation and prematurity, women need to weigh up carefully the possible advantage to the baby of continuing to grow, albeit slowly, in the womb, and whether they feel their prematurely-delivered baby can withstand either the epidural or general anaesthetic which will be used and whether being taken out of the womb early can really be considered an advantage. If you do choose to have an elective caesarean, it may be better to have it done under epidural anaesthesia, as this has the advantage of relieving pain as well as lowering blood pressure. The decision whether or not to have an elective caesarean for pre-eclampsia is yours alone and should be made based on all the facts. In order to get all the facts you may have to go outside the hospital walls to organizations such as the PETS, AIMS and the NCT.

Anaemia
Very few women really suffer from anaemia during pregnancy. It is thought that the extra iron which the baby takes from the mother's system is offset by the fact that she is not losing blood from her monthly periods – at least in the first few months of pregnancy. The risk to the mother who is anaemic is that she is less able to cope with heavy bleeding, that her contractions may be more painful and less efficient and that she is more vulnerable to post-partum infection. For the baby it means that there is less oxygen in the blood, which can result in poor growth and premature labour.

The symptoms of anaemia are almost indistinguishable from the common symptoms of pregnancy and include tiredness, shortness of breath, dizzy spells and becoming easily exhausted after strenuous activity. The only way to tell for sure if you are anaemic is to have a blood test, and even then the results are open to wide interpretation.

Blood is made up mostly of red blood cells (erythrocytes) and plasma. The volume of white blood cells (leukocytes) and platelets, while equally important, is minute. Haemoglobin is the pigment in red blood cells which carries oxygen to the various parts of the body. Plasma is the colourless solution of proteins and salts in which the red and white blood cells are suspended. A non-pregnant woman is said to be anaemic if her haemoglobin levels fall in relation to her plasma levels. The problem with accurately diagnosing anaemia during pregnancy is that the volume of blood in a mother's body nearly doubles, and the greatest increase is in plasma levels. It is thought that an increase in plasma levels of up to 50 per cent is a normal adaptation to pregnancy. This occurs in response to the increased production of waste products, heat and sweat which must be carried to the kidneys and the skin and excreted. There is also an association between low levels of plasma and low birthweight, and it is thought that unusually high levels of haemoglobin in comparison to plasma are linked to pre-eclampsia.[17] Recent research has shown that women with low haemoglobin levels during pregnancy may actually give birth to bigger, healthier babies.[18]

During pregnancy the baby's needs take priority, so iron and other nutrients are first diverted to meet the baby's needs. If the mother's levels of iron are initially very low, it is she who will suffer. However, recent research shows that women's body chemistry changes throughout pregnancy to allow greater absorption of iron. At 36 weeks the body's ability to absorb iron is nine times greater than in early pregnancy.[19] This confirms that, given a good diet, the body is quite capable of keeping both mother and baby healthy during pregnancy.

In the light of this, taking supplements simply because you are pregnant may be an ill-judged reaction. The chemistry of your body is very delicately balanced, and before trying to pump up your iron levels artificially you should also consider the possible side-effects. Synthetic irons can cause constipation, nausea, dizziness and diarrhoea, and are less easily absorbed, placing greater strain on your body. Vomiting and diarrhoea can deplete the body's stores of iron, creating a vicious circle. Tonics with natural iron, such as Floradix, are better, though expensive (unless you can get them on prescription). If you are taking iron supplements you may need to take other supplements to help absorption, such as zinc and vitamin C. There is also an emotional and psychological side-effect of taking supplements. Once your doctor writes out a prescription for iron supplements, you become a patient whose general health is in question and who needs to be monitored. If you can't be bothered to pop all these pills, some simple changes in your diet may be all that are needed. Iron-rich foods such as pulses, grains, red meat, especially offal (preferably organic, as there can be toxins in kidneys and liver), shellfish such as clams and oysters, dried apricots and nuts, plenty of protein, B vitamins (especially B_{12}) and folic acid all help to create blood which is rich in iron and so rich in oxygen. Things which decrease iron supplies include excessive amounts of caffeine (tea, coffee, colas), a diet which is high in refined sugars and carbohydrates, smoking, drinking and drug taking.

Gestational Diabetes
Gestational diabetes could been dubbed, among other things, 'a collection of symptoms looking for a disease'. There is no doubt that a woman who has diabetes prior to becoming pregnant needs to have her blood sugar levels and her diet monitored carefully if she wishes to remain healthy, carry her baby to term and go into spontaneous labour. However, for women without diabetes, the search for gestational diabetes is more often an excuse for over-zealous practitioners to restrict women's diets and weight gain. A doctor may (erroneously) use the term gestational diabetes to explain the fact that a woman had produced a very large baby.

Lots of women produce large babies, and before a diagnosis of some vague pathology is made, practitioners should consider carefully other possible influences such as the birthweight of both parents, the woman's pre-pregnant weight and her weight gain during pregnancy, and whether or not the pregnancy might be post-term. Even though there is no clear definition of gestational diabetes, once diagnosed it places a woman in a 'high-risk' category, which will mean greater anxiety for her and more 'routine' tests which confer no benefit to her or her baby.[20]

It is hard to say with any certainty what 'normal' blood sugar levels are in pregnancy, though they are certainly different (higher) than in non-pregnant women. The reasons for performing a glucose-tolerance test in the first place are probably as good an indication of possible problems as the test itself. These include obesity, a previously large baby, a previous stillbirth or malformed baby. Also, the glucose intolerance test is notoriously unreliable. The same practitioner doing the same test twice on the same woman in the same ante-natal appointment will not be able to get the same results in as many as 70 per cent of cases.[21]

It is thought that a mother with unusually high blood sugar levels will produce a large baby who may itself have abnormally high blood sugar levels, and therefore may experience hypoglycaemia (a sudden drop in blood sugar levels) after birth. However, only about 30 per cent of babies weighing 4,000 g (8 lb 13 oz) or more actually have abnormally high glucose levels. You do not have to agree to have your newborn baby's blood sugar level tested – which involves removing a sample of blood – if you do not feel this is justified.

Placenta Praevia

Early pronouncements of placenta praevia – a condition where the placenta is lying over the cervix – are usually made on the basis of information gained from an ultrasound scan, and have no value. In early pregnancy many placentas appear to be lying low enough to constitute a risk of this condition. However, as the pregnancy progresses, in almost all cases the alleged risk never materializes.

A large Finnish study of 8,000 women, in which half were scanned between 16 and 20 weeks, revealed 250 in the scanned group to be at risk of placenta praevia. At delivery only four actually had this complication – and one of those was not detected by the scan. This means that 247 women were left to worry needlessly for the entire length of their pregnancies. In the non-scanned group there were also four cases of placenta praevia, all of which were diagnosed in labour. In all eight cases healthy babies were born by caesarean.[22]

The early diagnosis of placenta praevia does little more than create anxiety in the mother and prompt practitioners to schedule elective caesareans which are unnecessary.

Lifestyle

It is probably beyond the scope of this book to delve completely into the subject of healthy versus self-destructive lifestyles. Women who smoke, who drink, who take drugs and who eat compulsively and unselectively may have other problems which make simply stopping 'for the sake of the baby' very difficult. But these are the women who are most at risk of having babies whose growth in the womb and whose long-term health are most at risk. There will always be exceptions: the chain smoker who produces a 4,090-g (9-lb) baby, the heavy drinker who produces a genius, the drug-dependent woman whose baby has all its limbs and mental faculties. But on the whole we can't afford to kid ourselves: Healthy mothers make healthy babies.

Smoking

The effect of smoking during pregnancy has been the subject of extensive research. A study conducted by the Health Education Authority revealed that 89 per cent of women consider smoking to be dangerous for their babies.[23] Yet less than a third claim to quit during pregnancy. Something like 10 per cent actually smoke more during pregnancy. Of those who do quit, half will be smoking again within a month of the baby's birth.[24]

Smoking definitely reduces birthweight. On average the babies of smokers weigh 200 g (7 oz) less than those of non-smokers. Smoking has the same effect on the fetal vascular system as it does on the mother's vascular system, making it less efficient and depriving the baby of essential oxygen. There is a 30 per cent greater risk of stillbirth and perinatal death, a 27 per cent higher chance of miscarriage. Babies of smokers are four times more likely to succumb to sudden infant death syndrome (SIDS), and twice as likely to be born prematurely. Because women in poor socio-economic circumstances are the ones who are most likely to smoke and continue to smoke during pregnancy, their children can end up doubly disadvantaged. They may have to deal with long-term physical problems, such as breathing difficulties and allergies, as well as life in a disabling environment.[25] Younger mothers (under 25) are the ones who are most likely to be smokers. Since 40 per cent of babies are born to women under 25, the problem is potentially very widespread.

Smoking can make the unpleasant symptoms of pregnancy even more unpleasant and persistent. Mothers who smoke are more likely to experience vomiting, nausea, diarrhoea, urinary tract infections, thrush, bleeding and miscarriage. Unlike non-smokers, these symptoms for mothers who smoke do not generally get better during the second and third trimesters. Smokers tend to complain more about feeling unwell later in pregnancy.

It is recognized that smoking can be a coping strategy. Mothers who smoke may do so in order to maintain a fragile equilibrium in their lives from day to day. They may continue to smoke, in spite of being aware of the dangers to their babies, because they don't like to be dictated to by other people, because they disagree with warnings about the potential dangers and feel that 'it won't happen to me' or because smoking is the most positive means of dealing with daily hassles. If their partners smoke, it can make quitting even more difficult, requiring as it does a shift in behaviour and attitude on both their parts. Most of the advice doled out by practitioners in ante-natal clinics ignores all this, as well as the highly addictive nature of cigarettes. To some extent mothers who smoke are damned if they do and damned if they don't. If they continue to smoke they suffer the guilt and anxiety (which often makes them smoke more) from the thought that they might be damaging their unborn child. If they quit they may feel over-stressed and resentful. Stress, like smoking, is known to be a factor in women who produce low-birthweight babies.

As a means of encouraging women to stop smoking, many practitioners try to encourage smokers to reduce, initially, the number of cigarettes they smoke each day. One large study, however, has shown that there is no demonstrable benefit in reducing consumption in terms of increasing birthweight. Only quitting produces this effect.[26]

Women who smoke end up in hospital with hypertension and suspected intrauterine growth retardation more often during late pregnancy than those who don't. Unfortunately, a stay in hospital does not always help. One study showed that women confined to a hospital bed actually smoked more due to boredom and stress than if they had been at home.[27]

The good news is that, once you do quit, your body is capable of ridding itself of the noxious by-products of smoking quite rapidly. The most successful strategies which can help women quit smoking are those which help alter behavioural patterns. These include identifying the times, situations and places where a woman smokes and altering the pattern. For instance, if you smoke because you get bored, then it's time to get active – take a walk, paint the baby's room, cook, clean, iron, sew the button back on that shirt – anything which keeps your hands active. If smoking is a way to unwind and mark the end of work and the beginning of leisure, take a swim or an exercise class instead. If you smoke when you are watching TV or on the phone, keep alternatives such as chewing gum or a mixture of nuts and raisins handy. Special rewards can also help. Get together with a few other women who want to quit and support and congratulate each other. Use the money you have saved from not buying cigarettes to buy yourself one big special treat near the end of your pregnancy, or to buy little treats at the end of each week to help keep your morale up. This kind of behaviour-modification can help you get over the difficult first few weeks. After that it gets a little easier.

Drinking
There is no established 'safe' level of drinking during pregnancy. While it is generally accepted that a glass or two of wine a week will not cause undue harm, there has simply not been enough research to prove this to be true. Drinking can affect your baby at any time during your pregnancy because it crosses the placenta and gets into the fetal bloodstream fairly quickly. However, drinking during conception and the first trimester of your

pregnancy does the most damage. It is known that a single massive exposure to alcohol, or binge drinking, causes more harm than a little at a time.

Women who drink during pregnancy are usually given advice which includes monitoring the number of 'units' of alcohol they consume each week. The units system is based on the idea that one unit equals any one of the following: a half pint of ordinary beer or cider, a quarter pint of strong beer or lager, one small glass of wine, one single measure of spirits, or one small glass of sherry equals. Less than 10 of these measures in a week and you are classed as a 'social drinker' and the chances that you will harm your baby are very slight. More than 10 of these measures in any one week puts you into the 'heavy drinker' category, and you could be damaging your baby. When you are reliant on alcohol and unable to control how much you drink at any time, you are alcohol-dependent.

These categories are, of course, quite arbitrary and do not take into account things like a woman's lifestyle or her weight (a woman who weighs 75 kg [12 stone] is not going to be as affected by a unit of alcohol as one who weighs 45 kg [7 st]). It is also difficult to separate the effects of alcohol consumption from other factors such as smoking, socio-economic status, diet and race (for instance, black women who are alcohol-dependent seem to be more likely than other women to give birth to an affected baby).

The risk of directly harming your baby through alcohol consumption varies according to how much you drink. One study showed that women who drink 1 oz (equivalent to an eggcup) a day run only a very small risk. Those who drink $^2/_3$ of a bottle of wine a day have a 1 in 100 chance of harming their babies. Those who drink a bottle or more than four cocktails a day are increasing the risk to 1 in 5.[28]

The pattern of damage is well established. Damage to the heart, liver, kidneys and lungs is most likely in the first trimester, especially between 3 weeks (when the umbilical cord begins to form) and 8 weeks (when organ development is more or less

The Ante-natal Routine

complete). Inhibition of fetal growth occurs throughout the second and third trimesters.

The babies of women who are alcohol-dependent are the most at risk. They will not grow well and are likely to end up with Fetal Alcohol Syndrome, which in turn leads to a greater risk of cerebral palsy in the baby. Fetal Alcohol Syndrome is not as well defined as it might be, but the likely consequences include physical anomalies such as a short upturned nose, receding forehead, small eyes, asymmetrical ears, under-developed chin and cleft palate. In addition, the child may suffer mental retardation and cognitive, visual and hearing disabilities.

The best advice is to avoid drinking if at all possible while you are pregnant. The occasional drink may help you relax, but it confers absolutely no benefit on your baby; it may even be harmful. If you smoke and drink, the risk of a growth-retarded baby is increased fourfold.

The majority of women appear to reduce their alcohol consumption voluntarily without any help or advice.[29] For those who drink heavily and those who are alcohol-dependent, being able to talk to someone in confidence and getting the facts about the effects of alcohol on the baby can result in a reduction of around 10 per cent.[30] This may involve as little time as 15 to 20 minutes in consultation with your practitioner, helping you to identify the times and places where you are most likely to drink and giving you advice on how to modify your behaviour. You may be given the number of local or national support groups, which can be of great benefit. You may also want to try the ever-growing selection of alcohol-free wines and beers on the market now. If your partner is a heavy drinker as well, it may be of benefit for you both to speak to your practitioner, as it can be very difficult to reduce your drinking or quit altogether if your partner does not do the same.

Diet

To ensure a healthy baby, pregnant women should have a good diet. Unfortunately, around one third of the babies born in

Britain are born into families who are defined as 'poor' – those who are wholly or partially dependent on benefits or those whose income is less than half the average wage. In these families the food budget is severely reduced, as money which might have gone on food gets diverted to meet the bills. If a mother in these circumstances has other children, she may sacrifice her own food so her children can eat.

It is not just that good food is expensive. Some of the most nutritious foods are quite cheap. But in the West our own tastes and diets have become so distorted that it can be difficult to retrain ourselves to eat properly. A family which has been brought up on fried foods and refined sugars may find it very difficult to switch to pulses, whole grains and fresh fruit and vegetables. A mother within that family may find it very difficult to change her own habits.

Sometimes it is a problem of living in an area where there are only a few shops stocking only convenience foods. The effects of poverty, stress and lifestyle are also reflected in a woman's attitude to food. For a woman living in a disabling environment there may not be enough money, but also she may not have the energy to organize, shop for and prepare good food. As in all areas of maternal health, strong, practical support (from family, friends and professionals) can be the first step towards changing self-destructive habits.

Women also need to be aware of the way in which outside influences conspire to keep them from eating well during pregnancy. For many, diet is negatively linked with weight gain. In a culture which encourages women to stay slim, gaining weight in pregnancy can be a frightening thing. A poor diet in pregnancy isn't necessarily the result of not being able to afford good food. It may be the result of a fear of 'getting fat', worrying about your attractiveness, or an unconscious unwillingness to make the step into full-bodied motherhood.

Some of these stereotypes end up being reinforced by our carers. Midwives, as women, are prey to the same pressures. Those who are not at ease with their own bodies may end up projecting this onto the mothers in their care, recommending restrictive diets, or tut-tutting every time a woman gets on the scales. Male doctors may never have examined their own attitudes to women's bodies in pregnancy. They may unconsciously advise restricting food, salt and liquids in an attempt to keep their 'girls' looking good. They may not go so far as to advise a woman to *lose* weight. Instead they may 'innocently' recommend that she just doesn't put on any more! This confers no benefit to mothers – even those who are overweight before conception – or their babies.

A good diet benefits both mother and baby. Physiologically it is quite normal for the baby's needs to take priority over the mother's. Essential nutrients will be diverted first to the baby and then to the mother. If the mother is on a moderately inadequate diet the baby may be fine, but she may feel increasingly tired and unwell.

If the mother is on a very poor or restrictive diet it can have detrimental effects on the baby – chief among which is poor fetal growth. One guide concludes that 'During famine, mean birth-weight can be depressed by as much as 550 g (1 lb 3 oz), and iatrogenic [medical] dietary manipulation and restriction can have almost as marked an effect ... there can be no justification for allowing pregnant women to go hungry, or for imposing dietary restriction or major manipulation of the dietary constituents upon them.'[31]

The human body, however, is not a machine. It is not simply a matter of putting the right fuel in to keep it running smoothly. In general, a good daily diet should be made up of around 40 per cent cereal foods, 25 per cent vegetables, 30 per cent proteins and 5 per cent fresh and dried fruit.[32] Common sense dictates that you should avoid refined and processed foods, in particular those which have a high sugar content, spicy and fatty foods, foods with lots of additives (especially nitrates and flavour enhancers such as monosodium glutamate, or MSG), too much red meat, and stimulants such as coffee, tea, cocoa and cola (all of which contain caffeine). But every woman's tastes and appetites will be different. Certainly no woman should be forced to eat something she doesn't enjoy simply because it is good for the baby.

For some women, pregnancy is the one time in their lives when they can really enjoy food without feeling guilty. In this respect it can be a turning point in their lives. It can be a time when they finally realize that the ground will not open up and swallow them and lightning will not strike them dead if they eat and enjoy and put on a few pounds. What's more, for a mother who chooses to breastfeed, a good diet is essential if she is not to become run down. Establishing good eating habits during pregnancy will help give her the head start she needs to give her baby the best possible start in life.

General Issues in Ante-natal Care

Many pregnant women experience a steep learning curve during the nine short months their baby is inside them. Apart from the endless round of tests and procedures which they are subjected to, there are choices to be made about what to read, what classes if any to attend, whether or not you want to know your baby's sex, and whose dates are 'right' – yours or the doctor's (they are often different). For those who hold their own case notes, there's the challenge of trying to decipher the indecipherable. In addition, you may have to learn a whole new language – 'medicalese'. At first some of these things may seem either overwhelming or simply too trivial to be bothered with, but learning about them can be a crucial factor in getting the best possible care for you and your baby.

Ante-natal Classes

Ante-natal classes were devised to help fill the information gap. What a doctor or midwife couldn't or wouldn't tell a mother was expected to be passed on via the ante-natal class or group. Whether these classes live up to this expectation still remains to be seen. For women desirous of ante-natal education there is a wide range of choices, from the standard hospital

The Ante-natal Routine

class to classes run by groups such as the NCT and the Active Birth movement.

Natural birth pioneer Michel Odent has argued that interventions have caused women to 'forget' how to give birth.[33] This is also true of women in the West. However, I would certainly contend that what women have forgotten is not simply how to give birth – after all, it is what our bodies are built for and we have carried the knowledge of how to give birth deep inside us since the beginning of time. What women seem to have lost is a way of accessing this knowledge and of finding some sense of their relevance and potential as birth-givers. Ante-natal classes, which are ideally placed to reverse this trend, often do little to help.

The women who attended the first ante-natal classes were generally well-educated, middle-class women – those who were least likely to need constant attention. Today it is much the same. Historically women from less affluent and less educated backgrounds are reluctant to attend, preferring to rely instead on instruction from people they trust such as their mothers, grandmothers, sisters, friends and neighbours.

It may also be that the idea of ante-natal education actually appeals more to busy career-women – the ones who plan their lives and believe in avoiding unexpected surprises. But whatever the reason, ante-natal education has failed on many levels to deliver what is needed to the women who perhaps need it most.

Ante-natal classes are offered in hospitals and community clinics as well as by independent lay childbirth educators such as those in the NCT. The classes which you attend at the hospital or clinic exist primarily to explain the labour policy of that particular hospital. So, if the session is focused on labour, you will be shown the labour ward and the special care baby unit. You may be invited to examine some of the instruments used in labour, such as the amniohook, the epidural infuser, the electronic fetal monitor belt, forceps and ventouse suction cup. You will be given a list of the methods of pain relief which are most commonly used in the hospital, and some instruction in breathing techniques and relaxation. If it is a 'parentcraft' class the focus will be on how to take care of yourself and your baby after the birth. But whether they are teaching you how to cope with pain or to be a perfect parent, the message is still the same: 'You don't know how to do this, so we are going to teach you.'

Ante-natal classes are generally scheduled quite late in pregnancy, from 30 weeks onwards. By this time most women have already read the books, talked to their friends and found out for themselves much of what they needed to know about pregnancy and birth. A bit of creative thought applied to the issue of ante-natal education might reveal the logic of, and the real need for, classes or groups which meet throughout pregnancy, starting early on when women have the most questions and feel the most emotionally vulnerable.

Mothers would benefit from mixing with other mothers at all stages of pregnancy, as well as with those women who have already given birth. The fact that the content of ante-natal classes, and their timing, are determined by teachers and experts, has ultimately helped women to become more isolated from each other and to lose the ability to share the experience of pregnancy and childbirth in a positive way.

The ante-natal 'programme' at Michel Odent's hospital in Pithiviers, France, provided one kind of progressive model. There, different activities on different days of the week included the standard tour of the maternity ward, informal gatherings of mothers and mothers-to-be, yoga, singing and discussion of postnatal care.

Of the informal gatherings Odent has written: 'There was no moderator and no set program. People walk around and talk freely among themselves. Mothers holding their babies meet mothers-to-be – always a fruitful encounter.' The singing nights, which may sound strange to the reserved British personality, also reaped benefits: breaking down inhibitions, strengthening diaphragm muscles and helping women to concentrate on breathing out, all helpful for labour. In addition, 'other members of the family get to see the birth place: children are invited to sing with us and sometimes grandparents come, too. The warmth of these evenings is difficult to convey ... When we all sing together, the usual separateness between consumer and professional dissolves, a new relationship emerges.'[34]

Sadly, we in Britain are nowhere near this ideal. We have made very little progress towards improving either the quality of ante-natal education as an important and relevant social experience for mothers or the range and accuracy of the information given out during these encounters.

You do not have to attend any ante-natal classes if you do not want to. You have the right to shop around and to seek out alternative groups to those offered by your local hospital or clinic. You can even start your own group, not to educate but to communicate with other women, if you feel up to it. While there is evidence to suggest that women who are 'prepared' have an easier time of it in labour, it also begs the question 'prepared for what?' A woman who expects to be monitored, drugged and cut open may have an easier time accepting these interventions in labour, but may feel unexpectedly distressed by their after-effects. A woman who is prepared, in the inner sense of having confidence in her own birthing skill, may not only have an easier labour, but a happier time after her baby is born.

Birth Plans

Birth plans are the inevitable result of the failure of 'experts' and mothers to communicate with and trust each other. For years medical practice has been justified by insisting that women 'never asked for anything different'. Women, on the other hand, have insisted for years that they *have* asked, but have not been heard. However it evolved, until things improve it looks like the birth plan is here to stay.

A mother once revealed to me that her doctor had opined that he could always tell what the outcome of a birth would be by the content of a woman's birth plan: The more detailed it was, the more likely it was that he would end up doing an emergency caesarean. This displays a cynicism of the highest order and also fails to take into account the doctor's own, unconscious 'sabotage mechanism' – in other words, his own feelings that it would 'serve her right' if the assertive woman somehow 'failed'.[35] In spite of the widespread use of birth plans, some practitioners actively resent women being involved in their ante-natal care and births to this degree.[36]

The single most important point about birth plans is simply, *don't paint yourself into a corner with them*. Leave yourself room to respond to the way that your individual pregnancy and labour progress. It's easy to fall into the trap of believing that once you have made a birth plan you must stick to it come hell or high water. This is not the case. The word 'plan' is very misleading because it suggests a precise, military-like operation. Thinking in terms of a 'birth guideline' might be more helpful.

No one can plan for birth, not a GP, a midwife, an obstetrician or a mother. Your baby might surprise you by turning into an awkward position or taking longer to come than you expected (very common with first births). You may decide during labour that you wish to use some form of pain relief, but because you've written it down in your 'plan' that you didn't want any, you are left with feelings of having 'failed' in some way. Early in your pregnancy you may have envisaged your labour as a kind of an ongoing party with your partner, your best friend and half a dozen of your closest relatives by your side. Later on you may want something more private and will need to be able to change your mind with a clear conscience.

Birth guidelines are very valuable for letting other people know what you want, how you feel and what you are thinking. They are not, however, laws written in stone. You have the right to deviate from the plan or change your mind completely, in order that you may respond appropriately to your and your baby's individual needs during pregnancy and labour.

A birth plan should be written to express the things which are of the most importance to you during pregnancy and labour, but should generally include information on the following:

The Ante-natal Routine

* The place of birth.

* Your choice or birth partner(s); whether you would like your other children to be present (usually only possible at home births).

* Which ante-natal procedures you wish to have or avoid – e.g. ultrasound, the use of a Doppler to listen to the baby's heart – and what alternatives, if any, you propose.

* Which routine procedures in labour you wish to have or avoid – e.g. rupture of the membranes, fetal monitoring, induction, and any alternatives you may be able to suggest.

* How you would like the birth to be, in other words whether you would like to be mobile during labour, to eat and drink when you need to, what position(s) you would like to try and give birth in, whether you wish to have an unhurried second stage, whether you wish to labour and/or give birth in water, etc.

* How you feel about pain relief and what alternatives to conventional drugs you might wish to use.

* How you would like the third stage of your labour to go, i.e. do you want to deliver your placenta naturally and wait until the umbilical cord stops pulsating before it is cut, or would you prefer to have an injection of syntometrine, in which case the cord must be cut beforehand.

* Whether you are willing to be attended by students ante-natally and/or in labour.

* Whether you wish to hold and/or nurse your baby immediately after delivery, and whether you wish to have

* A request that any 'emergency' interventions are explained to you fully and your consent sought before they are implemented.

* Whether you agree to vitamin K being administered to your baby after birth, and if so whether by mouth or intramuscular injection.

* Your decision to breastfeed or not and, if so, instructions regarding whether or not your baby should be given water or supplemental feeds while in hospital.

* You may also want to consider what you would do if for any reason your baby needed to be taken into special care, i.e. would you still want to breastfeed?

Of course, you do not have to make a birth plan at all. But if you do you should also make your beliefs and emotional needs clear in it, as these are an important part of any birth. You can amend your birth plan at any time during your pregnancy or labour if necessary. You have the right to expect that if you have prepared a birth plan, that the ideas in it will be respected and your suggestions followed as closely as possible by your carers.

EDDs

Estimated delivery dates are just that – *estimates*. On the whole fewer than 10 per cent of babies arrive on the day predicted by an EDD. Often the accuracy of these dates relies more on the ability of different practitioners to use those silly little wheel calculators than on the mother's ability to determine the date of conception and count 266 days forward.

There have been numerous studies which show how inaccurate most methods of determining EDDs are. When it comes to

The Ante-natal Routine

the use of obstetric wheels it has been found that, when compared with the 280-day 'gold standard' calculation (counting 280 days from the last menstrual period) some 11 per cent were out by three or more days, and as many as 5.5 per cent were more than a week out.[37] The wheels, it was found, were badly printed and often the design was so substandard that the numbers on the inner and outer parts of the wheel did not line up properly, making it impossible to tell which date the arrow on the inner wheel was pointing to.

Many practitioners prefer to use the routine 12- to 16-week ultrasound scan to establish, in their minds and for the records, the baby's age. There is little evidence that this is significantly more accurate than any other method. Some practitioners have called for all GPs and midwives to stop 'confusing' women and tell them simply to ignore their own dates in favour of scan dates.[38] But this has more to do with sorting out the chaos in ante-natal clinics than it does with the presumed chaos in mothers' minds. Overall, the argument that women (and practitioners) should work within a given range of dates instead of a specific date of delivery[39] seems to be the simplest way of addressing everyone's concern about when the baby is due.

It may seem, early in your pregnancy, that this whole issue is trivial. But awareness of how inaccurate EDDs can be becomes increasingly important later on.

The rising rate of elective caesareans and inductions means we need to look very carefully at the possibility that we are hauling our babies out into the world before their lungs, kidneys, livers and digestive systems are ready to function independently. How can we be sure that a baby who is born by elective caesarean at 38 weeks isn't actually 36 weeks old? At the moment there is no one who can put hand on heart and say there is no lasting damage from taking a baby out of the womb early and depriving it of four weeks growth inside its mother.

It also creates emotional debate when babies are born prematurely. Can we be sure that a baby born, for example, at 22 weeks according to the doctor's calculation, and therefore not considered to be 'viable' (worth saving) under health service guidelines, isn't actually 24 weeks (and therefore 'viable')? Too heavy a reliance on EDDs can end up causing all kinds of problems. The vast majority of babies come when they are ready to come. This is not some perverse part of their nature, but a survival mechanism which assures that, under ideal conditions, children are not born before they can survive and *thrive* outside the womb.

You have the right to expect that your own dates, if you are confident of them and if they differ significantly from the hospital's, should be given priority if an elective delivery such as a caesarean or an induction is suggested to you for whatever reason.

Your Baby's Sex
Many hospitals make it their standard policy never to reveal the sex of a baby to its parents – unless there is a chance of gender-related disorders, in which case parents must have this information. This policy is enforced, it is said, in order to avoid litigation should the information be wrong, and to discourage the selective abortion of female fetuses. Some of the procedures and tests which are performed on women, such as ultrasound and amniocentesis, may reveal the sex of your baby to the practitioner. While ultrasound is not a very reliable indicator of the sex of your baby, amniocentesis usually is. Your doctor cannot reasonably withhold information about your baby once it has been gained. If you really want to know and you request this information, it should be given to you. If your practitioner refuses, you can, in the case of a result via amniocentesis, ask for the address of the laboratory which assessed your sample and write directly to it. The lab must give you the information. There is nothing in medical law or codes of ethics which gives a doctor the right to withhold this information – it is simply an exercise in power over the mother and an example of tackling a very specific problem from the wrong end. The aborting of female fetuses is a legitimate problem among some ethnic groups, and if practitioners are really worried about it then it is counselling for some, not denial of rights to all, which is the way forward.

The Ante-natal Routine

Case Notes

In several hospitals and clinics throughout the UK, women are now holding their own case notes. Case notes are different from appointment or co-operation cards, which also contain notes in a more abbreviated form. Your case notes are what the doctor or midwife writes about you in the hospital records. The possibility of 'allowing' a woman access to her own case notes is often presented as some kind of a gift. It is not. The Access to Health Records Act of 1990 makes it quite clear that from November 1, 1991, every patient has the right to have copies of his or her own case notes. Some practitioners still object to this, perhaps because they often write things of a most personal or derogatory nature. Greater access to our own case notes may prevent this and see the end of women who persistently ask questions being labelled as 'difficult', 'obstructive' or even 'neurotic', or women who show a certain ambivalence early in pregnancy being labelled as 'depressive'.

Even more disturbing, though, is the revelation that in cases where there has been a problem during the pregnancy or during labour, case notes have a tendency to 'disappear'. One study showed that women who had bad birth outcomes – stillbirths, babies with low APGAR scores, low-birthweight babies, preterm babies, etc. – were the ones most likely to be told that their case notes were missing or lost.[40] In the light of this possibility the best advice is, if you do hold your own case notes, make copies, and if you don't, get hold of them sooner rather than later.

On your case notes or co-operation card you will see certain abbreviations. This is what they mean:

Para 0 – This is a first baby
Para 1 (2, 3, etc.) – This is the first (second, etc.) birth
Para 1 + 1 – The mother has had one baby plus one miscarriage (or termination) before 24 weeks
LMP – Last menstrual period
EDD/EDC – Expected date of delivery or expected date of confinement. This is an estimate only. You could safely go into

spontaneous labour between two weeks before and two weeks after this date.

NAD – Nothing abnormal detected.

Alb – Albumen or protein in urine. In combination with high blood pressure and oedema, a possible sign of pre-eclampsia. Ideally there should be no protein in your urine, but sometimes there is, particularly in late pregnancy, without it signifying problems.

PET – Pre-eclamptic toxaemia – another name for pre-eclampsia or toxaemia.

Hb – Haemoglobin – the oxygen-carrying substance in your blood. Usually followed by a percentage. Lower than 10.5 may indicate that you need to supplement your iron intake.

Fe – The abbreviation for iron. Means that you have been prescribed iron tablets. Should be followed by a number indicating the strength of tablets prescribed, or an indication of advice such as 'take an iron tonic twice daily'.

Bp – Blood pressure. followed by your most recent reading, e.g. 120/80 (*see also page 129*).

FMF – Fetal movement felt.

FH/FHH/FHNH – Fetal heart/fetal heart heard/fetal heart not heard.

Oedema – Swelling, particularly in face, hands, ankles, feet and possibly vulva. Caused by fluid retention. Some swelling is common in late pregnancy. Excessive, sudden swelling combined with raised blood pressure may indicate pre-eclampsia.

Fundus – The top of the uterus. Measurement of the height of the fundus is used to check fetal growth.

Vx – The baby is presenting in the vertex – head down – position, the most common position.

Ceph – Cephalic – a different way of saying the baby is head-down.

Br – Breech – the baby is presenting bottom or feet first. At 32 weeks some 5 per cent of babies are breech. Most turn into the vertex position before labour.

The Ante-natal Routine

LOA/ROA/LOP/ROP – Left (right) occipito anterior or left (right) occipito posterior. All these refer to the baby's position in relation to the mother's body. The occiput is one of the bones in the baby's skull, the orientation of which – front (anterior), back (posterior), turned to the left or right – is described in relation to the mother's spine. Left occipito anterior is the most common position.

Eng/E – Engaged. In first pregnancies the baby's head usually engages some time in the last six weeks. In subsequent pregnancies the baby's head often doesn't engage at all until labour.

T – Term. An indication that you have reached your EDD. Fewer than 10 per cent of babies are born on this date.

Some hospitals are implementing the use of 'smart cards'. Instead of notes, mothers carry a plastic card, no bigger than a credit card, which is capable of storing, in electronic form, all the information about a mother and her pregnancy. Unfortunately they cannot be read without the use of a special machine, so they make the idea of 'access' to one's notes something of a nonsense. If you are a part of one of these schemes, you have the right, under the Data Protection Act 1987, to have a print-out of these and any other computerized records the hospital may hold on you. If your hospital uses both computerized and written notes, you have the right to copies of both.

It is assumed by many that a woman carrying her own case notes will be better informed about her care. To some extent that depends on who is making the notes and how well he or she shares and interprets what is being written down. Some 12 per cent of note-carrying mothers in one study at a large London teaching hospital felt that they had been 'not at all well informed', compared with only 1 per cent of card-carrying mothers.[41] This may mean that some practitioners use women carrying their own case notes as an excuse not to talk to them in depth about their ante-natal care.

In addition, the same study found a huge discrepancy between mothers' expectations and their experience of information-sharing.

Every Woman's BirthRights

A first questionnaire given to mothers on their booking visit asked how confident mothers were about the possibility of discussing their preferences and worries with medical staff – over 50 per cent anticipated no difficulty, and an even greater number, 75 per cent, anticipated it would be easy to talk about these things to a midwife. But at 32 weeks only 10 per cent had managed to discuss their preferences and worries with their practitioners.

During the course of your pregnancy and for 40 days after the last recorded entry in your notes, you can obtain copies of your case notes for the price of photocopying and postage. After that you can be asked to pay a statutory administration fee *not exceeding* £10, plus the cost of photocopying and postage. The hospital can suggest that you have someone there to help interpret the medical shorthand in your records. You do not have to agree, though some might find it helpful. You do not have to give a reason why you want access to your records and, barring the presence of any information about you or your baby's condition which the consultant feels would upset you (a ludicrous loop-hole in the law), he cannot refuse to let you see them. Some hospitals ask you to prove who you are by having a known and respectable person in the community countersign your application for access. This is mere bureaucracy. Any reasonable proof of your identity should be acceptable, such as having your application counter-signed by someone who knows you (a friend or employer, for instance), and you should certainly not have to pay out extra money to have your identity confirmed by a commissioner of oaths.

If you had a baby prior to November 1, 1991 and you wish to get hold of your medical records (perhaps you are pregnant again and would like to know more about what happened to you last time), getting your records can be a bit hit and miss. Some hospitals willingly supply them, others require you to get a solicitor to write to the hospital and request your records on your behalf. No reasonable request for access should be denied, though the cost will vary from hospital to hospital depending on how and where the records are now stored.

Medical Language

Medical language, in both its written and spoken form, can be a mystery. A woman will talk to many different practitioners during her ante-natal care, so it's as well to be prepared. Medical language is impersonal and impenetrable. It defines a woman in ways which are alien, even threatening. If this is your first baby you will be *nullipara* or *primigravida*. Worse, if you are over 30 you'll be a *geriatric* or *elderly primigravida*. If this is your second or subsequent baby you are *multiparous*. Your baby is an *embryo* for the first 12 weeks and a *fetus* thereafter. Your womb doesn't just get bigger, it acquires a *fundus*. You don't simply get swollen ankles and fingers, you become *oedemic*. It then becomes almost impossible to express yourself as a whole person experiencing a *life event* when you have been effectively carved up into unrelated pieces – a cervix, a birth canal, a womb, breasts, nipples, fetus and placenta – which are being taken over by a *medical process*.

Doctors know, albeit unconsciously, that to control the language is to control the process.[42] On the whole women have not done much to challenge this philosophy (in the context of their relationships with doctors or other figures of 'masculine' authority). This is in spite of the fact that we are the ones who conceive, carry and bear children. Because of our biology we are in a much more authoritative position to reconstruct the language of childbirth in a way that not only has the personal resonance and emotional impact which befits such a momentous event, but that also has everyday meaning to us as well.

When we talk about birth, might we just as easily say, and insist that those who attend us say, *baby* instead of *fetus*; *expansions* (of the cervix) instead of *contractions* (of the uterus), *birth* instead of *delivery*, *managing* (labour, pain, etc.) instead of *coping* (with labour, pain, etc.). We could, as childbirth educator Andrea Robertson has observed, insist that phrases like *'failure to progress'*, *'expected date of delivery'* and *'we lost the baby'* become *'a pause in labour'*, *'approximate birth date'* and *'the baby died'*.[43] What changes might occur if we were to stop talking in terms of *controlling* (anything) during labour and instead thought in terms of *allowing*?

The technical language of childbirth has no advantages for women, but many for doctors. It depersonalizes, and maybe more crucially desexualizes, a highly personal and sexual activity. It protects doctors and other carers from their own emotions, particularly their distress at seeing suffering or pain, and serves as a kind of shorthand which oils the machinery of the hospital environment. It is also an effective form of persuasion – medical language carries with it authority, weight and a greater sense of urgency, and can be used as a means of 'encouraging' women to agree to a procedure when everyday language fails to produce the desired result. Finally, it reinforces the idea that pregnancy and birth are mysterious and only fully understood by the experts.

In first pregnancies it is especially easy to be mesmerized into silence by the ceaseless routine which exists around pregnant women. Sometimes it will be the first time a woman has ever been to a hospital; the realization that she can't just have a baby without all the fuss can be quite shocking. Even a normally confident, assertive woman can be thrown by the powerful presence of a consultant and the efficient atmosphere of a hospital or clinic.

In addition, women and doctors come from two different worlds and use language in very different ways. In any consulting room it's not just a mother and a doctor – two people with two different sets of experiences – it's often a man and a woman – two sexes which have been socialized to use language in different ways (even female doctors can use medical language in a very 'masculine' way).[44]

For a doctor the purpose of a consultation is to diagnose, to impart selective information, to assert status. It is an exercise in power and an opportunity to show that while he is an expert in obstetric and gynaecological medicine he is emotionally independent from any impact it may have on women.

For a woman, the same consultation may well be an opportunity to seek reassurance, but that is not all. It is also a chance to discuss options and share the impact of impending motherhood on her life, to gain information, ask questions and feel a sense of solidarity with her carer.

Many doctors are adept at the reassurance part. It is the part of their job which makes them feel the most benevolent. Doctors often bestow 'good' news about the baby as if it were a gift, reinforcing the idea that a healthy baby is somehow a result of their good care and attention instead of the mother's.

The information part is less of a success story. Studies have shown that women consistently fail to get the information they desire from practitioners. Obstetricians, in particular, tend to underestimate the amount of information which mothers want. In one study of the interactions between mothers and obstetricians, it was revealed that while some 84 per cent of mothers want, for instance, to know about the possibility that their baby is deformed, only 21 per cent of obstetricians consider this important information. Similarly, only 14 per cent of obstetricians believe that women would like to know about books to read, but 70 per cent of women reported they wanted this information. The study concluded that in general most mothers 'fail to obtain all the information they would like to obtain from their obstetricians, even after many antenatal visits'.[45]

Often doctors avoid giving out information because, they say, they don't want to confuse or alarm a woman. They dislike being 'prodded' for information because they see it as a challenge to their authority. This kind of intractable position can destroy any possibility of effective communication between mothers and doctors.

As uncomfortable as it may be initially to change the way we relate to our care-givers, we must remember that we have the right to have our needs for more information and consideration taken seriously. It behoves us to assert that right, not as a means of bullying or controlling our practitioners, but as a means of communicating what we want and expect from them.

4
Testing, Testing

It's common for pregnant women to feel confused about the reasoning behind, and the results of, some of the tests on offer to them. It's just as common not to be aware of the difference between screening tests and diagnostic tests. Most of the routine tests are done for *screening* purposes only. This means that they cannot tell you definitively whether there is anything wrong with you or your baby, but can give you and your practitioner a good idea of whether there is a chance that you or your baby *may* be at risk of developing complications ante-natally or in labour, or whether there might be anything wrong with your baby.

Because the vast majority of mothers and babies are perfectly normal and healthy, the screening tests done early in your pregnancy are used mainly to provide a useful baseline, or yardstick, against which the results of any further tests administered throughout your pregnancy can be measured. Deviation from this baseline might mean that something is amiss, but this is rarely the case. For instance it is quite normal for blood pressure to fluctuate, particularly late in pregnancy; and some women do get traces of protein and glucose in their urine as well as swollen ankles and fingers, without this indicating pre-eclampsia or glucose intolerance. Pregnancy places a degree of strain on a woman's body, and her body responds by constantly adjusting itself to increasing hormone levels, weight and the rearrangement of internal organs as the baby grows.

No test is 100 per cent accurate, and as many as 25 per cent of women, at either end of the scale, end up with either *'false positive'* results – indicating there is something wrong with the baby when there isn't – or *'false negative'* results – indicating that there is nothing wrong with the baby when, in fact, there is.

Diagnostic tests are usually offered to women who have been identified as being at risk of pregnancy complications or of carrying a baby who is in some way ill or handicapped. It is important to remember that diagnosis does not necessarily guarantee a cure. For instance, tests to assess the mother's health may reveal conditions which can be 'corrected' during pregnancy. However, with tests performed to assess the baby's health, should they reveal an abnormality often the only 'positive' step to 'correct' the condition is termination. It is the rising rates of obstetric terminations of abnormal fetuses, rather than some vague magic worked by obstetric technology, which is responsible for today's low rates of babies born with abnormalities.

What is more, ante-natal testing is often very impersonal and performed in an atmosphere of clinical efficiency by people with little or no communication skills. This can make a mother feel very anxious and insignificant, and may even prevent her from asking necessary questions. For some, increased anxiety can increase the risk of developing complications ante-natally and in labour. You do not have to have any ante-natal testing if you do not want to. If you do, it may be to your advantage to explore all the possibilities and alternatives first.

Routine Screening

The ante-natal routine commences at your initial, or booking visit. For the majority of women their first step will be a visit to the GP to report or confirm that they are pregnant and to give a detailed history of themselves and their partners, if the doctor doesn't already have this. Most women go to this appointment alone, but if your partner can go with you, provided you have discussed your options and preferences with each other beforehand, you may find it helps you to say what you want and to feel supported. These days, home pregnancy testing kits are so accurate that many GPs do not insist that you take a further 'official' test, especially if the results of your home test are very obviously positive. However, some GPs still like to have a woman's pregnancy 'scientifically' confirmed – which means that they will take a sample of urine, exactly as you did at home, and stick a plastic stick into it, exactly as you did at home.

Overall, letting your GP or midwife know you are pregnant, sooner rather than later, is a reasonable thing to do. This way, if you wish, you can have all the basic screening tests done and weigh up the need for any further, special diagnostic tests in your own time. If you want to or if it looks likely that you should have any of the diagnostic tests available, for instance, to check for Down's Syndrome, Spina Bifida or any other congenital abnormalities, these tests must be done early in your pregnancy, usually before 18 weeks.

If you have chosen to book directly with a midwife you should contact the Supervisor of Midwives at your local hospital. She can either come to your home for your booking visit (a convenience usually reserved for women having a home birth or those who have disabilities which prevent them from getting to the clinic) or you will be invited to attend a local clinic or hospital. But whomever you book with, the initial visit and the antenatal routine will be the same.

Blood Test
A sample of blood will be taken from you during your booking visit. This will be used to confirm your blood group and Rhesus status. If you are Rhesus positive your blood contains something called the Rhesus factor; if you are Rhesus negative it does not. A

Rhesus negative mother with a Rhesus positive baby will be offered an Anti-D immunization within 72 hours of giving birth to ensure that any subsequent children are not afflicted with Rhesus disease (that is, where the mother's body, as a result of the inevitable exchange of red blood cells between mother and baby during pregnancy and birth, produces antibodies to the Rhesus factor. These antibodies will vigorously attack the blood of any subsequent Rhesus positive babies, producing jaundice, anaemia and, in some cases, brain damage and death). The exchange of red blood cells across the placenta in first pregnancies is nominal and unlikely to result in damage to the baby, but some centres administer Anti-D prophylactically (meaning just in case, as a preventative measure) to mothers anyway.

The same sample of blood will also be tested for signs of anaemia and for immunization against Rubella (or German Measles). If you are not immune to Rubella you will be offered a postnatal immunization and will be advised to limit your contact with children who are likely to be infected, as Rubella, while a relatively mild disease for mothers, can cause abnormalities in the baby she is carrying if contracted before 15 weeks. In addition your blood sample will be tested for venereal disease, viral hepatitis (or Hepatitis B), and possibly diabetes. Some hospitals also test for HIV if you are likely to have a higher than average chance of having the virus (such as if you have had many lovers, are a drug user, if you have a bisexual partner or if you have had a blood transfusion in the last 20 years).

The results of the HIV test, if positive and assuming you wish to continue the pregnancy, will, in theory, be confidential and kept separate from the rest of your notes; staff will not normally be informed until you are in labour (when it has implications for their health as well as the health of the baby). In practice, though, the only way to ensure confidentiality is to have your baby at home, away from the hospital grapevine.

Urine Test

Your urine will be checked initially and at every subsequent ante-natal visit. At each visit you will be given a clean sample bottle in which to bring along to your next visit a 'mid-stream' sample of urine. To get a mid-stream sample, first allow a little urine to pass out of you, thus reducing the possibility that protein from your vagina will mix with the urine sample and give a false reading. Then allow an amount of urine to go into the sample bottle. You don't need to fill it, a sample small enough to dip a paper stick into is all that's required.

Urine is mainly checked for sugar, protein, ketones and blood, for the presence of urinary tract infections such as cystitis, and for kidney infection. Changes in the composition of your urine are quite common during pregnancy and may vary depending on factors such as what you have eaten and how much stress you are under. However, sudden, significant rises in sugar or protein may indicate glucose intolerance or pre-eclampsia. If you feel particularly concerned you can test your own urine at home by purchasing Uristix from your local chemist.

Blood Pressure

Your blood pressure will be checked every visit to check for the possibility of hypertension (raised blood pressure) or incipient pre-eclampsia. What your doctor or midwife is looking for is sudden deviations, either up or down. Your blood pressure reading consists of two different sets of figures. The top number is your *systolic* reading, the bottom one is your *diastolic* reading. Systolic pressure can change at any time depending on whether you have been running around or whether you are under stress. It is changes in your diastolic reading which are important, as these could indicate there are problems. Having said that, it is normal for your blood pressure to rise a little during the late stages of pregnancy anyway. There is no such thing as 'normal' blood pressure. In practice anything between a lower limit of 90/50 and upper limit of 130/80 is 'normal'. Your own blood pressure may vary for any number of reasons, so small differences from visit to visit are no reason to hit the panic button.

If you arrive at the clinic late and/or feel flustered and upset for whatever reason, this may affect your blood pressure. Some women who dislike being in a medical environment are prone to 'white coat hypertension'. Take a few minutes to rest and calm down, then ask your practitioner to take your blood pressure again.

Weight
Chances are you will be weighed at each visit as a means of assessing your baby's growth. Many observers are now questioning this practice, not simply because of the demoralizing effect it has on so many women, but because maternal weight gain does not always follow a predictable curve and is therefore an unreliable method of assessing fetal growth (or lack of it). After all, we have all known women who have put on 18 kg (3 st) and have given birth to 2750-g (6-lb) babies, and other women who have barely put on 6 kg (1 st) and have given birth to 4100-g (9-lb) bruisers. In the light of this, more progressive clinics are abandoning the ritual weighing of mothers.

The routine of 'popping on the scales' has to some extent become a substitute for assessing a mother's general state of health and the baby's growth by simply looking at her and feeling her abdomen. Also because women's weight is such an emotive subject and because every practitioner has his or her own different, often prejudicial views about how 'fat' or how 'thin' a pregnant woman should be, mothers are often subjected to advice which is humiliating, conflicting and sometimes dangerous. Providing everything else is OK, your weight gain is your business and not subject to the 'permission' of your doctor or midwife (however, if you suddenly gain or lose a lot of weight you should tell your practitioner, as this could be a sign of pre-eclampsia or some other complication). If you feel sensitive about your weight, you can request not to be weighed.

Abdominal Palpation

This is a simple, hands-on procedure in which the doctor or midwife feels around your abdomen to ascertain the height of the fundus (top of the uterus) and check that it coincides with the estimate of how far along your pregnancy is. Later on in your pregnancy, abdominal palpation can be used, with varying degrees of success, to assess how much amniotic fluid there is, how big the baby is and which position the baby is lying in. Measuring the abdomen from the pubic bone to the top of the uterus is a fairly effective way of assessing fetal growth and age, though in the age of ultrasound many practitioners have lost this skill.

Vaginal Examination

These are becoming more rare in pregnancy as there is very little evidence that they are really necessary or fulfil any useful function. There are still some doctors who wish to perform them as a fail-safe to confirm a pregnancy and assess how far along it is, as well as to judge pelvic proportions. Many women find internal examinations unpleasant; you have the right to refuse one if offered or advised. If you decide to have one there should be a nurse or midwife present. Many doctors abuse this ethical guideline or make their women patients feel neurotic for asking for a nurse or midwife to be there. You have the right to insist without being made to feel bad or as if you are wasting everybody's time.

Some doctors and midwives leave it until around the 36th week of pregnancy to suggest an internal examination. There may be slightly more sound reasoning behind this, as by then it will be easier to assess correctly your true pelvic proportions in relation to the size of your baby. Having said that, if checking your pelvis is the only reason for an internal examination you can probably do without it. Women have an amazing knack of making babies just the right size to come out of their bodies. If this were not the case our species would have died out long ago! If you do have an internal examination and it hurts – speak up. Many doctors dismiss women's complaints that the examination hurts with the reassurance that they should 'relax' or 'breathe deeply' or 'not be so sensitive'. This is probably because most doctors learn to perform internals on plastic dummies or on women who are unconscious and can't give permission or complain (the ethics of which are *highly* questionable). A properly performed vaginal examination should not hurt *at all*. If it does, it is the practitioner's lack of skill and not the woman's sensitivity which is at fault.

Fetal Heart Monitoring
Your baby's heartbeat will be checked at each visit. This can be done with a simple stethoscope, a Pinard (or ear trumpet), or a Doppler (or sonic aid). A skilled midwife should have no trouble finding your baby's heartbeat with the stethoscope or Pinard, however it is fast becoming standard practice to use the Doppler. There is no doubt that the first time you hear that little heart going like the clappers it can be thrilling. Unfortunately, sonic aids use small quantities of ultrasound to detect and magnify the sound of the baby's heart, and we need to weigh up the thrill with the possible side-effects of repeatedly exposing our babies to this largely unevaluated technology.

Whatever method is used, to some extent the results still rely on the skill of the practitioner. I can remember, on several occasions, lying belly exposed on the examination table while an embarrassed doctor prodded me with the sonic aid trying to find my baby's heartbeat without success. Had I known then about the questionable safety of ultrasound and the possibility that the sound was painful to my baby's sensitive ears, I would not have allowed this to continue. Any mother has the right to refuse the use of a sonic aid. If you wish to hear your baby's heartbeat and you don't want the Doppler used, ask your practitioner to use a stethoscope and let you listen that way.

Ultrasound
The enthusiasm with which the medical profession has embraced ultrasound has given rise to the following joke:

Enthusiast: 'Ultrasound is the answer'
Sceptic: 'Yes, but what was the question?'

Ultrasound should not be used routinely, but it is. Mothers tend to get scanned at least twice: once in early pregnancy (16 to 20 weeks) to detect abnormalities and establish the baby's age and where the placenta is, and in later pregnancy (32 to 36 weeks) to detect intrauterine growth retardation. It is increasingly used to detect fetal abnormalities, for which, given an experienced operator, it has a fairly high success rate. It is one of the most widely used and at the same time most under-evaluated technologies used in the ante-natal routine.

To perform an ultrasound your practitioner will spread a gel over your tummy (don't wear your best clothes!). The purpose of this is to provide a smooth area for the scanner to move over. Often women are asked to drink a pint of water before the scan. This is generally only necessary if the scan is performed before 12 weeks. Early in pregnancy, when your uterus is still relatively small, it can be difficult to get a good picture. A full bladder pushes the uterus up into the abdomen, allowing the person performing the scan to get a better picture. There is absolutely no need to have a full bladder later in pregnancy. In fact, a full bladder in late pregnancy can distort the image and make the placenta appear to be lying lower than it actually is. Many women, unaware of this, have suffered enormous discomfort for no reason at all. If your practitioner asks you to drink lots of water before a late scan it is likely to be out of habit rather than because of any sound medical reasoning. You can always refuse, or ignore, this request.

While there is some evidence to support the view that selective use of ultrasound in high-risk women can be of benefit, there is none to suggest that its routine use has any value at all. An editorial in the *Lancet* – the Bible of the medical profession – determined that:

> Published work on the biological effects of ultrasound imaging is surprisingly thin. There have been some reports

of adverse effects in fetal animals and damage to cells in culture, but the data are seriously deficient and many questions have simply not been addressed. There have been no randomized controlled trials of adequate size to assess whether there are adverse effects on growth and development of children exposed in utero to ultrasound. Indeed, the necessary studies to ascertain safety may never be done, *because of lack of interest in such research* [my emphasis].[1]

This statement, made 12 years ago, is still true. Since that time, however, there have been some major studies done on the diagnostic efficacy of ultrasound which have given rise to the view that there is no medical reason to propose a routine ultrasound scan to some 80 per cent of the population of pregnant women.[2]

Unfortunately, medical confidence in ultrasound has been so infectious that many women don't feel that they have been 'properly' cared for ante-natally unless they have one or two (or more) scans. At the same time, those who advise caution where ultrasound is concerned are seen as killjoys, and those mothers who choose to reject routine scanning are viewed as being negligent and foolhardy. Enthusiasts believe that a scan confirms the 'reality' of the baby to its mother, that it reduces maternal anxiety and increases confidence. In addition, the ultrasound scan has given rise to an obsession with 'prenatal bonding'. These days the photographs (and videotapes offered by some hospitals) of the first scan have become almost as big an event as the birth itself.

Scans are not 100 per cent accurate – a fact which is ignored by most enthusiasts. Much of the accuracy of the scan depends on the ability of the person carrying it out to interpret what he or she sees. Many mothers assume that for a person to use an ultrasound machine he or she must have received adequate training. This is not always the case. Although practitioners can obtain a Diploma in Medical Ultrasound from the Society and College of Radiographers, not all do – and there is no legal requirement for them to do so.

Any practitioner can purchase a scanner, and any practitioner can use one. As a result, ultrasound scans are performed by doctors, midwives, radiographers, sonographers and students. Often their training has consisted of watching colleagues use the machine until they feel confident enough themselves to 'have a go'. Many GPs have purchased scanners and use them on their women patients having received only the most rudimentary instruction.

Even more worrying is the fact that there are no strict standards relating to the frequency output of ultrasound equipment (those standards which do exist allow for a huge variation in output levels). To obtain an image on the screen, ultrasound uses high-frequency sound waves, which are then directed at an object – in this case the baby. These sound waves bounce off solid objects, and the resulting 'echo' returned to the computer produces a picture.

The frequencies which mothers and babies are subjected to vary wildly depending not only on the output of the machine, but also on other factors such as the amount of body fat on the mother (fat absorbs some of the ultrasonic waves) and the strength of the magnification the operator is using (higher magnification means higher output). The length of time an examination takes can also vary. A usual time given is around a quarter of an hour, but again, this is only a guide. That pleasant sonographer who takes a great deal of time and trouble showing interested parents every tiny little finger and toe is also increasing the amount of exposure the baby gets; at the moment no one can say with any certainty whether this can be regarded as safe.

Nuchal Scan
This type of scan is performed very early (11 to 13 weeks). The results of the scan are combined with your age to calculate your risk factor for Down's Syndrome and other chromosomal abnormalities. What the sonographer is looking at is the nuchal fold at the back of the baby's head. When the fold is especially thick, it appears on the screen as a large black space behind the baby's neck. This is thought to be an indication of abnormality. Because

the scan is performed so early, it is potentially more risky for the baby. This procedure cannot give you a definitive answer about your baby's health, however it is less invasive than other procedures such as amniocentesis and, since it appears to be reasonably accurate, may initially prove a better course of action if you are worried about your baby's health.

Transvaginal Scan

Also known as intravaginal ultrasound, this is a relatively new technique. Many practitioners are excited by the supposedly clearer pictures which it gives, but consumer and feminist groups admit to being uncomfortable with the concept. The transvaginal probe is often described by doctors, who wish to allay women's anxieties, as no different from a tampon or a speculum. Actually it is more like a dildo.

It is a plastic cylinder 10 to 15 cm (4 to 6 inches) long which is covered with a condom before being inserted into the vagina. Once inserted it is pushed in and out and moved from side to side until the practitioner gets the desired picture. The overtly sexual nature of the probe, plus the fact that it exposes the baby to a greater amount of high-frequency sound while at the same time denying it the protection of its mother's abdomen and amniotic fluid (which would normally absorb some of the ultrasonic waves) has led many to voice their concerns.

There is also an increased risk of infection with this method, as the condoms have been known to break. This method also brings with it an increased, though uncommon, incidence of sexual abuse. There have already been several cases in Australia and the US which have led to the coining of the phrase 'diagnostic rape'. If your doctor suggests a transvaginal ultrasound examination, first find out why he feels this is necessary and what he feels he could see with this probe which he could not see with a conventional scanner. He should have a very good reason. If you decide to have a transvaginal ultrasound, there should be a midwife or nurse present. If there isn't you can refuse to allow the doctor to proceed.

Some Possible Side-effects of Ultrasound

What we don't know about ultrasound far outweighs what we do. Because of this the evidence of harmful side-effects, however slight, should not be ignored. It's as well to remember that mothers were routinely subjected to X-rays for nearly 50 years, all the while being told that it was perfectly safe, until a flood of research proved it to be causing an increase in childhood cancer. The development, use of and research into ultrasound has in many ways paralleled that of the X-ray.

Repeated ultrasound exposure increases the chance of miscarriage and has also been shown to double the chance of premature labour.[3,4] It has also been linked to intrauterine growth retardation.[5]

There is evidence that the APGAR score of babies repeatedly exposed to ultrasound is lower, though this has not been linked to any long-term problems.[6] However, studies on animals have suggested possible damage to the baby's immune system as well as neurological and behavioural abnormalities. Experiments with guinea pigs showed that Doppler ultrasound raised the temperature of brain tissue close to the bone by as much as 5.2°C (41°F).[7] Since first scans take place at around 16 weeks, when the developing brain is most vulnerable, it has been reasoned that vital cells may be damaged or destroyed with 'little prospect of replacement', resulting in long-term neurological damage.[8] When the increased incidence of left-handedness,[9] the tendency towards dyslexia,[10] and speech delay[11] are mentioned, many doctors simply shrug it off. Yet these are functions controlled by the brain, adding fuel to the argument that ultrasound does alter neurological functions in ways which we have not yet begun to explore.

A phenomenon which is currently being monitored, if only anecdotally at the moment, is known as 'jumping babies'.[12] Many mothers assume that the wiggling and 'dancing' their babies do during an ultrasound or Doppler examination is a sign of normal activity. However, as much as 20 years ago researchers believed that these 'jumping babies' were actually responding in pain and distress to the high-frequency sound produced by the scan.

There have been some shocking cases recently which illustrate the hit-and-miss quality of ultrasound examinations. At one hospital in Cardiff several women were diagnosed as having dead babies and told they must have a termination, only to find out, just before the procedure, that actually their babies were alive and well.[13] One woman went through this ordeal in *both* of her pregnancies. These women suffered indescribable emotional and psychological distress at the hands of inexperienced (and sometimes just thoughtless) staff using, more often than not, old and faulty equipment. A recent report on the findings of a large trial in West Yorkshire revealed that 1 in 200 babies terminated because of abnormalities detected by ultrasound was, in fact, perfectly normal. It also showed that in 1 out of every 100 cases of ultrasound failed to detect significant handicaps for which mothers should have been offered a termination.[14]

If an ultrasound examination reveals something wrong with your baby, you have the right to insist on a second scan performed by a different operator (preferably a senior radiologist) on a different machine. Often a woman requesting this will be told there's no point, because there is no doubt about the diagnosis. You do not have to accept this. Many hospitals routinely perform a second scan to confirm the diagnosis before performing a termination. There is no reason why this second scan can't be performed immediately (as opposed to three or four days later). If your partner is with you let him or her do the talking for you. If not, don't be afraid to be pushy, make a nuisance of yourself and raise your voice if you need to – under certain circumstances your baby's life could depend on it.

Choosing or Refusing Ultrasound
You have the right to refuse any or all ultrasound examinations, especially those which are suggested merely as routine. You can ask for and should receive a full explanation for any scan which is suggested for a specific purpose. If you choose not to have any ultrasound scans but still wish to have some record of your baby's growth recorded in your notes, you can ask for your

practitioner to make a record of the fundal height at each visit. This is a perfectly reasonable method of monitoring your baby's growth.

If you choose to have one or more scans – and most mothers will – then there are certain things which it may benefit you to know first.

You should ask your practitioner early on for the ultrasound statistics from wherever you will have your scan. You can ask how many scans are done in theory and in practice (a hospital may have an ante-natal plan which includes two scans, while in practice a significant number of mothers may wind up having four 'routine' scans); talking to other mothers may provide you with the most accurate picture. You can decide independently how many scans you wish to have. It is probably wise not to have any scan before 12 weeks, as this is when the greatest tissue damage is thought to occur, and to ask that a record of your ultrasound exposure, even if it is often mere guesswork, is kept and attached to your case notes. This should include dates, exposure times, and the calibration of the machine. You may be doing your daughters and granddaughters a considerable favour by insisting that practitioners keep more careful and professional records of these routine exposures.

You might want to ask for the screen to be tilted your way. Even if you don't understand all that you see, it sends a signal that you are not simply a passive recipient of the procedure. Always ask the operator what he or she is looking at or for. Some hospitals' or local policies prohibit sonographers from discussing what they see on the screen in any detail, so the information you get may be very general and inconclusive. However, the more women ask questions, the more pressure it puts on the medical establishment to remember who is serving whom.

Take someone with you. While your partner has no legal right to be there, most hospitals accept that he (it is always assumed it will be a he) has a moral right to be present. Some are so rooted in the idea that a mother will want to bring her male partner that they do not allow female partners to be present. This, of course, discriminates against single mothers, lesbian couples and those whose partners cannot or will not attend for whatever reason. If your doctor is very keen that you should have an ultrasound, you could turn this to your advantage by refusing unless the partner of your choice is allowed to be with you.

Advantages:

* There are no advantages to the *routine* use of ultrasound.

* It has fewer proven side-effects than amniocentesis or CVS (Chorionic Villus Sampling) and in skilled hands it can be used to detect Down's Syndrome and a significant number of congenital abnormalities accurately.

* Some practitioners (and some parents) feel scans establish an early bond between mother and baby.

* It is a necessary part of amniocentesis and CVS procedures, helping to guide the needle safely into the womb.

* It can be used to confirm an ongoing pregnancy after a heavy bleed.

* During the first three months of pregnancy, ultrasound can give an accurate idea of the baby's age. This is useful only for women who are unsure of their dates.

Disadvantages:

* Ultrasound is an unevaluated technology.

* Use of frequent ultrasound has been linked with intrauterine growth retardation.

* For some women it doubles the risk of premature labour and miscarriage.

* There is evidence that ultrasound has a negative effect on neurological function, producing more left-handed babies and children with dyslexia and delayed speech.

* There is almost no way of knowing what frequency you have been exposed to – your operator may not even know. Pulsed Doppler ultrasound uses a higher frequency than real-time machines and external fetal heart-rate monitors.

* Early scans – before 12 weeks – are thought to cause the most cell and tissue damage.

* Ultrasound is an invasive procedure for the baby – its shrill sound can be heard by the baby, causing pain and distress.

* Diagnosis of certain conditions, such as placenta praevia, are inaccurate 95 per cent of the time.

* After 25 weeks ultrasound is wildly inaccurate in determining fetal maturity.

* The heat produced by ultrasound in brain tissue which is close to bone can cause irreparable cell damage.

AFP/Double/Triple Test

There are many different types of screening tests which can be done from a single blood sample to calculate a woman's potential risk of having a baby with neural tube defects, Down's Syndrome and other chromosomal abnormalities. These tests look for chemicals, known as 'markers', in the blood. The number of markers the test is looking for is indicated in the name of the test. Because it is relatively non-invasive and there is no risk of miscarriage, many women will agree to these tests, looking for reassurance and thinking they have nothing to lose. In fact they have a great deal to lose, because the tests' high 'false positive' rate (indicating there is something wrong when there isn't) means that women spend a significant proportion of their pregnancies worrying about whether they are carrying an affected baby, only to find out after a cascade of other tests that there was nothing to worry about in the first place.

There is very little counselling given to women on the implications of a positive result, and what exists is often confusing. One GP related his experience of his wife's counselling this way. In this excerpt the doctor is explaining about the estimated risk factor, which is the result of the triple test:

Jo: What do you mean 'estimated'?

Senior registrar: Well, for every 57 women under the age of 37 who test positive, only one will in fact be carrying a Down's Syndrome child.

Me: And 56 will go through the emotional hell and amniocentesis for no reason.

Senior registrar: Exactly. That's why I wouldn't touch it.

Jo: If it's positive, would I automatically have an amnio?

Senior registrar: Tricky. You're a late booker ...

Me: That's not our fault.

Senior registrar: So if you had an amnio you'd be too late for a termination by the time the results are back.

Jo: So I'd have CVS or fetal blood sampling instead?

Senior registrar: You could do, yes. But remember, the risk of induced abortion from these procedures is double that for amnio.

Me: What if the test was positive and we did nothing?

Senior registrar: You'd still have a 56 out of 57 chance of a normal baby.

Jo: What if the test was negative?

Senior registrar: You could still have a Down's Syndrome child. At best the test only picks up 50 per cent of cases. And you had an early bleed, which can elevate your AFP and render the test useless.

Me: What do other patients say when you tell them all this?

Senior registrar: Usually I don't get the chance. They have the test and only realize the implications if a positive result comes back. Then most of them say they wish they'd never had it done in the first place. Do you still want it?

Jo: I'm not sure.

Since the father of this baby was both present *and* a GP, this conversation was more of a professional courtesy than a routine explanation. But as the author suggests, 'if two doctors have trouble getting their heads around the ramifications of a triple test, what hope have other patients got?'[16]

The AFP, or alphafetoprotein, blood test is usually performed at around 16 to 20 weeks and is not the same as a routine blood test. AFP is produced by all human fetuses. If there is an open neural tube defect, AFP 'leaks' out into the amniotic fluid and the mother's blood. This is why high levels of AFP are associated with a greater risk of open neural tube defects such as Spina Bifida and anencephaly. Low levels of AFP are associated with Down's Syndrome. The AFP test is not very accurate and, generally speaking, it is used to weed out mothers who will then go on to have further tests (amniocentesis, scans, etc.). Only 10 per cent of mothers who are diagnosed as having raised APF levels in their blood, and who subsequently go on to have amniocentesis, have affected babies. The results of the test are combined with the mother's age to calculate her individual risk factor.

In reality, there is a wide range of 'normal' levels of AFP, all of which can be influenced by outside factors. Alphafetoprotein levels can vary from day to day, and in the second half of pregnancy they double approximately every four weeks. So, if you are further along than estimated this will show as a high reading. This is also true in the case of multiple pregnancies. Inaccurate dates and multiple pregnancies account for about a quarter of raised AFP levels.[17] If you had an early threatened miscarriage, if you smoke, have viral hepatitis or if you are black you are also more likely to have raised AFP levels. The sex of your baby also has an impact. Boys produce slightly higher levels of AFP, though not enough to alter test results significantly. If you are very overweight or insulin-dependent, this can push levels down.

A woman is generally thought to have a positive result if her individual risk of having an affected baby is 1 in 250. This standard cut-off point is used in all screening tests and has evolved from the use of amniocentesis, because this is the point at which the odds of having an affected baby are finally greater than the odds for a miscarriage caused by the procedure (though of course there is no risk of miscarriage with blood tests). AFP testing continues to be used, however, because women who screen positive will automatically be advised to have amniocentesis. The wisdom of this, however, is currently being questioned since an experienced ultrasound operator can pick up suspected abnormalities just as accurately and without the proven risk of miscarriage which amniocentesis carries. The arbitrariness of the risk factor is illustrated by the fact that if a woman has a 1 in 251 risk factor she is told there is nothing wrong with her baby. If she has a 1 in 249 risk factor she is told her baby may be abnormal!

In theory, the more markers which the test looks for, the greater its sensitivity – that is, its ability to detect accurately the possibility of abnormalities. The double test, which looks for raised levels of alphafetoprotein and lowered levels of unconjugated oestriol, is mostly redundant now. In its place is the triple test which looks, in addition to these, for raised levels of total human chorionic gonadotrophin (HCG). This is now pretty much the gold standard of screening tests.

If you don't feel confident in the results of your test you can ask for it to be done again. In most hospitals women who screen positive are re-tested as a matter of course. Chances are that the second test will give completely different results. These tests are sometimes performed with the proviso that the mother agrees to terminate an abnormal baby. This is highly immoral. No doctor has the power to force you to terminate your pregnancy, nor can a doctor deny you a test or withhold information about your baby on the grounds that you have not agreed to an abortion. Even if you do initially agree to abort a baby with suspected handicaps, you have the right to change your mind when the results of the test are confirmed. Women who show raised AFP concentrations have a much higher risk of spontaneous miscarriage before 20 weeks, so there is a chance that a badly affected baby will be aborted naturally before the doctor can do the job medically. This 'act of nature' may be easier for the mother to accept. All these things should be borne in mind if the test is offered to you.

Advantages:

* Because the test can be performed on blood samples it is relatively non-invasive and carries no physical side-effects.

* Results are available quickly, usually within a week.

Disadvantages:

* The AFP and triple tests are not very accurate. At best they only detect 50 per cent of affected fetuses.

* A high false-positive rate (between 5 and 10 per cent) means that many mothers will experience the anxiety of further tests and long periods of uncertainty about their babies' welfare – for no reason at all.

* Tables used to calculate a mother's individual risk factor do not take into account all the variables which can raise or lower the levels of the various markers in her blood.

* To most practitioners it is 'just another blood test' and so there is very little counselling given to women about its accuracy and the implications of a positive result.

* A negative result is no guarantee that your baby will be born without abnormalities.

Diagnostic Tests

When considering whether or not to have a diagnostic test, you must first try to weigh up your own 'risk factors' against the 'risk factors' of the individual test. Unfortunately, many of the variables which go into calculating a woman's risk factor, though quite nebulous, can end up being applied in a very black-and-white way, resulting in some unbelievably narrow parameters for defining 'low risk'. For instance, a woman is considered to be at risk if she is, among other things: under 18 or over 36; if she is having her first child or has had four or more children; if she is uncertain of the date of her last menstrual period; if she has had a previous small baby or a previous large baby; if she has had a previous caesarean; if she has had a previous long labour or a previous short labour; if she has had a previous forceps delivery; if she is overweight before conception or is underweight before conception; if she is too short (under 150 cm/5 ft); and if she has put on too much or too little weight during pregnancy.

Sometimes practitioners can become so absorbed in the mechanical process of determining a woman's 'risk' factor that they forget to look up from their theoretical charts. The calculation of a woman's individual 'risk' factor via a series of pre-set questions should never take the place of clinical judgement based on the individual who is sitting right in front of the doctor or midwife. Otherwise too many normal and healthy women end up being assigned to the 'high-risk' category, with all the attendant emotional, physiological and mental trauma that this label brings. In fact, only between 10 and 30 per cent of women allocated to high-risk groups actually experience the adverse outcomes of which the scoring system declares them to be at risk.[15]

Amniocentesis
This is a diagnostic test which is generally performed in the second trimester of your pregnancy, between 16 and 22 weeks, when it is thought there is enough amniotic fluid to allow enough to be drawn off for testing without causing too much

harm to the baby. The fluid which is withdrawn can be analysed in two different ways depending on what your practitioner is looking for. First, the amniotic fluid can be checked for levels of AFP and thus the possibility of neural tube defects such as Spina Bifida. In addition, cells from the baby's skin which are floating around in the amniotic fluid can be cultured (grown) to check for chromosomal abnormalities such as Down's Syndrome.

By the time a mother gets to this stage she may already have had two AFP or triple tests, a couple of scans and possibly even a CVS (Chorionic Villus Sampling – *see page 152*), where either the procedure or the culture has failed. Emotionally and spiritually she will be very vulnerable. Add to this the fact that the results of an amniocentesis take anywhere from two to four weeks to come back, meaning that a termination if necessary will take place at a very late stage, and you have all the ingredients for a very stressful pregnancy.

In response to this, some institutions offer 'early' amniocentesis. This is defined as being performed before 15 weeks – sometimes as early as 9 weeks. This is often presented to mothers as a safer alternative to first-trimester CVS. What mothers are generally not told is that, for older women in particular, early amnio carries a substantially increased risk of miscarriage. Women aged from 34 to 36 have twice the risk, and women aged 37 or over two and a half times the risk of experiencing a spontaneous abortion as a result of the procedure, than those of a similar age opting for traditional amniocentesis.[18]

Older mothers are in a double bind because they are statistically at a greater risk of having an affected baby but are also at greater risk from the procedure. Apart from an increased risk of miscarriage, early amniocentesis results in more leaks of amniotic fluid (2.9 per cent compared with 0.2 per cent) and more bleeding (1.9 per cent compared with 0.2 per cent).[19] Though most of these pregnancies will be carried to term and delivered without complications, the emotional strain which mothers are expected to bear should not be underestimated.

In order to perform the test your abdomen will be disinfected and, guided by an ultrasound picture, a long, thin needle will be passed through the skin, the abdominal muscle and the uterus into the amniotic sac. There is a 1 in 1,000 chance that the needle will miss its target and puncture a blood vessel or the placenta, or hit the baby instead. In these circumstances it will have to be withdrawn and the whole procedure performed again. Mothers are usually (and certainly should be) asked whether they would like the doctor to try again then and there or whether they would prefer to make another appointment. Under these circumstances it is usually best to schedule another appointment and give your body time to recover, even though the wait may seem agonizing.

Amniocentesis should NEVER be performed without the aid of a simultaneous ultrasound picture. This technique, known with good reason as 'blind' amniocentesis, carries a high risk of the needle puncturing, and withdrawing blood and tissue, from vital parts of your baby's body such as the internal organs and the brain. A number of hospitals in Britain still use this 'blind' technique. You do not have to agree to this procedure. You can ask to be referred to a large regional hospital where it is likely that operators do 100 to 200 each year, and are more skilled in the proper technique.

The risk of miscarriage is between 0.5 per cent and 2 per cent; if miscarriage occurs it is usually three or four days after the procedure. In skilled hands the risk of miscarriage can be reduced considerably, so if you are going to have this test make sure you go to a clinic where they do a lot of them. In the UK an operator is considered proficient if he or she has done around 50 procedures under supervision (unlike in Denmark, for instance, where operators have to do 200 under supervision before they are allowed to perform the test alone). Don't be afraid to ask how many procedures your doctor has done, and if you are not confident in his or her ability, ask that someone else perform the test.

After an amniocentesis a mother may experience uterine contractions which are strong enough to take her breath away, and there may be considerable leakage of amniotic fluid and some bleeding. There is an increased risk of infection. There is a 2 per cent chance that, due to culture failure, the test will have to be done again. This can result in an agonizing wait. Because abortion is never mentioned in genetic counselling, women are woefully misinformed about the different procedures used in early terminations – where the cervix is dilated and the contents of the womb sucked out – and late terminations – where labour is induced, usually with prostaglandin, and the mother 'gives birth' to the baby. The difference in the emotional impact of the two procedures is obvious.

Amniocentesis is a traumatic and invasive procedure. While it should not, and would not, be the first choice of many women, once you are on the runaway train of ante-natal screening your eventual destination is likely to be the outpatients' clinic for an amnio. Around 8.2 per cent of women are offered amniocentesis on the basis of their age alone; some practitioners have advocated testing all women over the age of 35 regardless of their perceived 'risk' factor. Although it is true, for instance, that the probability of having a Down's Syndrome child increases as a woman gets older, age alone is not a reliable indication of risk. For instance, a 38-year-old woman is currently advised that her overall age-related risk of having a Down's Syndrome baby is 1 in 140. But the actual risk can range anywhere from 1 in 10 to 1 in 10,000 depending on individual factors. In addition, research has shown that, while screening all women over the age of 35 would detect 100 per cent of Down's Syndrome babies in that age group, it would also prove to have been unnecessary for 99 out of every 100 women, and would expose them and their healthy babies to the risk of amniocentesis-related miscarriage.[20]

Practitioners are increasingly using AFP, double and triple tests to screen for those women who should go on to have amniocentesis. However, as mentioned (*see page 141*) these tests have a high false positive rate, so increasing the number of screening tests may not necessarily be the answer (particularly in view of the reported accuracy of the nuchal scan). The greater the number of these (or any) tests performed on the basis of age alone, the greater the number of 'low-risk' women being tested. This increases the number of variables that a practitioner would have to negotiate in order to arrive at a woman's individual risk factor, such as age, weight, lifestyle, ethnic group, whether the woman is insulin-dependent, whether her dates are correct and whether she is carrying a previously undetected twin (and remember, a practitioner need only make a small miscalculation to put a woman into the wrong risk category).

Amniocentesis can't guarantee that your baby will be perfect. There are more than 5,000 kinds of disorders, and each test can only eliminate the limited number of disorders which we currently look for. Equally, it cannot guarantee if, or the extent to which, your baby may be damaged. It is believed that, of those babies who are aborted on the basis that amniocentesis revealed raised AFP levels (and thus the possibility of neural tube defects), 6.5 per cent, had they been born, would have had no handicaps at all. Of those that had, 15 per cent would have had no open neural tube defects or only mild Spina Bifida, which would not have caused any problems.[21] In simple language this amounts to 1 in 5 'normal' babies which are mistakenly aborted.

Often the hospital will leave the decision about whether an autopsy (known as a 'histology' when performed on very tiny babies or uterine contents) should be performed. Sometimes in early terminations there is not much to examine, though it is unusual for there not to be enough to perform a chromosomal analysis. Many parents find not knowing for sure if their baby was abnormal the worst part. Others may feel, either for personal or religious reasons, that they would not like to know. If a histology is performed you have the right to know the results. You may like to have not just the obstetrician but also a paediatrician present when you go in to discuss the results of an autopsy or chromosomal assessment.

Very few women receive counselling before amniocentesis, and few practitioners actually feel confident about providing this essential service. Mothers need to know more than just their individual risk factors. They also need to know the risks of the test. If counselling is provided it is usually on the day of the test when the mother may be too anxious to take it all in. Your partner should be with you for any counselling sessions and you should ask to be counselled on a date prior to the test so that you can have a chance to think things through away from the hospital environment.

Advantages:

* Amniocentesis is reasonably accurate. It can correctly detect Down's Syndrome 90 per cent of the time, and neural tube defects 80 to 90 per cent of the time.

* It can be used in the third trimester to assess fetal lung development and whether the baby is likely to be born with respiratory distress syndrome (RDS).

* The test will reveal the sex of your baby. This is important for parents who carry sex-related disorders such as haemophilia or Duchenne muscular dystrophy.

Disadvantages:

* There is a risk of miscarriage of between 0.5 per cent and 2 per cent. This figure rises depending on how early the test is performed and how old the mother is.

* A negative result does not guarantee a healthy baby, since only a limited range of defects are screened for.

* Amniocentesis can be an uncomfortable experience with distressing side-effects such as leakage of amniotic fluid, bleeding, uterine contractions, and infection.

* In 1 out of every 1,000 cases the needle will miss the amniotic sac and puncture a blood vessel, the placenta, or

the baby instead. Under these circumstances the needle will have to be totally withdrawn and the procedure started again.

* Amniocentesis is safest when performed between 14 and 16 weeks. This is quite late, and the 2- to 6-week delay in getting results can mean that if termination is indicated it will happen quite late in the pregnancy. This can cause both physical and emotional trauma.

* There is a 1 in 200 chance that a baby whose mother has had amniocentesis will have either very low birthweight or neonatal respiratory problems.

* In 2 per cent of cases there is culture failure, which means that the test will have to be repeated.

* The safety of amniocentesis depends largely on the operator's experience.

Chorionic Villus Sampling
CVS has been widely used since the 1980s, and was originally hailed as the conquering hero of fetal abnormality tests until a large-scale European trial conducted by the Medical Research Council revealed that it led to more diagnoses of abnormality, and so more terminations, more spontaneous fetal deaths before 28 weeks, more neonatal deaths (because more babies were being born very immature), and longer hospital stays for newborns.[22]

This test, also known as placental biopsy, is used to diagnose the same things as amniocentesis, with the exception of Spina Bifida. It is given early (between 9 and 11 weeks) and, depending on where the placenta is lying, is performed either through the abdomen (transabdominal) or through the cervix (transcervical). The transabdominal route is a newer procedure with a lower failure rate and is associated with less bleeding afterwards – though most doctors still prefer to use the transcervical route, which they are more familiar with. In 10 to 25 per cent of cases the transcervical route will result in spotting or light bleeding.[23] In 4 to 5 per cent of cases the transcervical route will result in a sub-chorionic haematoma (a swollen area under what will eventually develop into the placenta, known at this stage as the chorion) which may be associated with bleeding. In up to 50 per cent of cases there may be fetomaternal haemorrhage (fetal blood leaking into the mother's system).[24] This can be the result of damage to the placenta, and if the mother is RH negative and her baby RH positive it can result in Rhesus isoimmunization (the mother's body producing antibodies which can attack the baby's blood, destroying some of its red blood cells and causing anaemia, jaundice and occasionally brain damage). Because of this some practitioners do not recommend this procedure for women who are Rhesus negative.

Either way, a scan will be used to locate the chorionic villi and a hollow needle or small tube will be inserted into the uterus. A small amount of tissue will be gently sucked up through it and, depending on the method of analysis, results can be obtained within a day or two. Your operator should be doing around 50 of these procedures each year to be considered competent.

There are many problems with CVS. First of all, the chorionic villi are part of the tissue which surrounds the embryo. They are like tiny 'roots' which will eventually implant themselves in the uterine wall and develop into the placenta. No one has yet assessed what removing part of the placenta at this early stage has on its growth and eventual efficiency. Not surprisingly, though, one of the side-effects of CVS is low-birthweight babies.

One of the most disturbing new findings regarding the safety of CVS is that tests performed before 9 weeks can result in missing limbs and limb deformities.[25] Because of this one study concluded that CVS was probably less safe and more prone to error than amniocentesis.[26] Others believe that, given an experienced operator, the safety of CVS is at least equal to that of amniocentesis. The fact that the medical profession cannot agree on something so basic as the safety of CVS should be enough to make mothers more cautious about accepting it.

One explanation for the greater detection of abnormality which CVS claims is that, because the test is performed so early, it is detecting fetuses which would have been spontaneously aborted before the second trimester, when the more traditional amniocentesis would be performed. In other words, we are detecting abnormalities and asking mothers to make the horrendous decision of terminating their pregnancies, when, if left to nature, the decision would have been taken out of their hands – and possibly easier to accept. One study found that women who miscarry after CVS experience a great deal of guilt and grief, and blame the loss on their own selfish desire to get an earlier result.[27] It may be that more social support and accurate information in early pregnancy would be a more effective and safer way to help allay women's fears that they are carrying an abnormal baby. Either that or we should all follow the example of Hassidic Jewish women and not turn up for ante-natal care before 26 weeks when it's too late to be put through the mill.

A CVS test can be carried out earlier than a traditional amniocentesis, but the risk of miscarriage is double that of amniocentesis. Doctors sometimes convince women to have the CVS test by telling them that it carries less of a risk than an *early* amniocentesis. In obstetrics there is a test to suit everyone, every new test is better than the last one, and we never find out the truth about the side-effects until the next 'better' test comes along.

Advantages:

✳ Preliminary results can be obtained between 24 and 48 hours after the test is taken, though some practitioners prefer to wait a week or so, by which time the full results are available.

* For mothers deemed to be at high risk of having a baby with abnormalities, the fact that CVS can be performed relatively early can be reassuring.

Disadvantages:

* There is a 2–4 per cent risk of miscarriage and evidence that, if performed too early (before $9^{1}/_{2}$ weeks), CVS can result in missing limbs and limb abnormalities, and facial deformities.

* Nobody knows what the possible side-effects of removing some of the vital placental tissue has on a child's long-term health.

* In around 2 per cent of cases some of the mother's cells get mixed up with the baby's, rendering the test inconclusive.

* There is up to a 6 per cent chance that the results will be inconclusive due to culture failure – three times that of amniocentesis.

* CVS may not be the end of the ordeal. Some 10 per cent of women who have CVS go on to have amniocentesis as well.

* CVS cultures are prone to ambiguous results (known as 'mosaicism') where some, but not all, of the culture from the same specimen shows signs of abnormality.

Pelvimetry
X-rays preceded ultrasound scans as a way of assessing fetal health. They were stopped because of the link between X-rays and childhood cancer. The link between X-rays and childhood cancer still exists. So if at all possible you should avoid any form of X-ray during pregnancy.

Your doctor knows this, but nevertheless women are offered pelvimetries (pelvic X-rays) to assess the size of the pelvic inlet and outlet.

There is something about the process of assessing the size of a woman's pelvis that is a little bizarre. History has proved that the vast majority of women have pelvises which are quite adequate to push a baby through – otherwise there would be no babies. The only point in history when women had small or deformed pelvises was during Victorian times when rickets were common and the growth of the pelvic bones could be stunted as a result.

Pelvimetries are actually so inaccurate that some hospitals are abandoning them altogether. Because the measurements we are dealing with are quite small (the average pelvic inlet measures around 10.5 cm (4 inches) and the average pelvic outlet measures around 12.5 cm (6 inches),[28] the interpretation of the X-ray need only be out by 0.5 to 1 cm (roughly a quarter of an inch) to place a woman in a 'high-risk' category.

At any rate it is impossible to predict how the pelvis will behave and what dimensions it will achieve in labour.[29] The only way to find out is to go into labour and see what happens. Suspected cephalopelvic disproportion (where the mother's pelvis is too small and/or the baby's head too big to permit a vaginal birth) can only be proved by a trial of labour. If your doctor offers you a pelvimetry the safest advice is to refuse politely but firmly. It will confer absolutely no benefit to either you or your baby.

Advantages:

✲ There are no proven advantages to pelvimetry.

Disadvantages:

✲ X-rays are known to be harmful to fetuses, resulting in an increased incidence of childhood cancers.

* The results of a pelvic X-ray are not an accurate indication of how the pelvis will respond in labour. Measurements of the pelvic inlet and outlet are estimates only and open to a wide range of interpretations by different operators.

* A bad result can by psychologically damaging – making a mother believe that she will not be able to deliver her baby.

Cordocentesis
Cordocentesis, also known as percutaneous umbilical blood sampling (PUBS) or fetal blood sampling, is a very fiddly procedure which should not be performed before 18 weeks and is generally only used to confirm the results of anther test. In order to take a sample of the fetal blood, a fine needle is inserted via the mother's abdomen into the point where the umbilical cord meets the placenta. The operator MUST use simultaneous ultrasound to site the needle correctly. This is a very delicate operation; the point which your practitioner is aiming for is less than half a centimetre (about an eighth of an inch) in size, so the potential for failure and damage is understandably huge. It is associated with an increase in placental and cord problems, and the rate of miscarriage after the procedure is between 1 and 2 per cent.

Getting Off the Conveyor Belt

When deciding about special tests, women don't just grapple with the endless sets of abstract percentages and risk scores. They grapple with the reality of their own lives, their values, emotions and perceptions of themselves. They also grapple with practical considerations – the money, time and energy it would take to raise a disabled child.

In theory, the best way to get off the conveyor belt of antenatal testing is not to get on it in the first place. But for some this can prove very difficult. Many women avoid acknowledging their pregnancies, to themselves or to others, until they have had the health and normalcy of the baby confirmed by an 'expert' with the aid of a test (or two or more). For them the time between confirming their pregnancy and the first scan or blood test can be filled with enormous anxiety.

Practitioners seldom understand that the process of deciding whether or not to have a test, and if so what test to have, is not always rational. For instance, women are usually asked to decide about testing at a time in their pregnancies when they do not feel well themselves and may be worried that this is a reflection of the baby's state of health. Nor is it acknowledged that the concepts of risk and imperfection may be viewed differently by mothers in different contexts. A young woman with an unplanned pregnancy, uncertain of who she is and whether or not she will make a life with the child's father, may be much less able to cope with the idea of an 'imperfect' baby than a woman in her mid- or late thirties who has other children, a secure relationship and a greater sense of herself. Also, as Caroline Flint, a midwife of vast experience, recalls, there is often no rational connection between the severity of the condition and a mother's sense of shock or grief: 'I remember the total rejection for several days of a baby girl because she had extra digits on each hand. I also remember the loving and gentle nursing of a baby with very severe Spina Bifida by her parents as she gasped her way through the few short days of her life.'[30]

In a culture which places such a high value on 'normality' and 'perfection', bonding with an imperfect baby can involve the painful process of acknowledging the imperfection in ourselves. Women, in particular, are more inclined to punish themselves for their imperfections, especially if those imperfections are connected to their bodies. Unconvinced that their less-than-perfect bodies could ever produce a perfect baby, some women enter into ante-natal testing as if it were a penance.

For others ante-natal testing is seen as a responsibility. They feel it is up to them to make sure that their children have the best chance in life. Increased knowledge of the harm which some tests can do means that they must now weigh up the benefits of these tests against their potential physical and psychological risks.

There are 5,000 different chromosomal anomalies – many of these seem to make no difference to a person's life, while others mean certain death. Tests like amniocentesis and CVS can at best pick up only a handful of these. You will need to be clear about what you do and don't want to know. If, for instance, a test turns up an anomaly about which we know nothing, will it benefit you to be told about it? Some mothers ask that they only be told about anomalies which are known to affect their children either physically or mentally. Otherwise, they reason, they might always be looking for signs that their child is different or abnormal, or they might be tempted to blame individual quirks in behaviour or personality on 'bad' chromosomes, causing anxiety and psychological damage in the process.

Ask yourself whose agenda you are following. Ante-natal testing benefits doctors as much, if not more, than women (though few would be willing to admit it). Detecting abnormal babies and terminating them protects them from their own distress at bringing a disabled or sick baby into the world. If a test reveals an abnormality which is incompatible with life, such as anencephaly or severe Spina Bifida, often there is great pressure brought to bear to terminate the pregnancy. For some parents this is the best option. For others there may be more to gain from allowing the pregnancy to take its course and to see their baby born, even if the baby will only live for a few hours or days.

There are no easy answers when it comes to ante-natal testing. No one can force you to accept a test if you do not want one. Neither can you be forced to terminate a disabled baby if you don't want to. Nor can you be made to follow some sort of timetable for making your decision. The choice is entirely yours and is probably best made in your own time, away from the hospital environment. Be led by your instincts and, above all, make sure that whatever decision you come to is yours and not your doctor's.

5

Managing Labour

The concept of actively managing birth has been around for 25 years or so. Using a mixture of pharmacological, instrumental and surgical interventions, it was conceived as a way of shortening labour, reducing pain, avoiding serious complications and improving outcomes. There has yet to be any evidence that it does any of these things. The single biggest impact which active management seems to have had on birth is that more caesareans than ever are being performed because of 'failure to progress'.

With active management, the uterus is seen as a mechanical, inanimate object which works on the simplistic principles of cause and effect. Given synthetic hormones which resemble those produced naturally in labour, the ineffective uterus will contract better and the troublesome cervix will simply yield. Having yielded, the baby can either be pushed out by the mother or extracted by the doctor – and voilà, you have a 'birth'.

In practice, of course, it is not that simple. From the practitioner's point of view there is no organ that is so uncontrolled and so erratically unpredictable as the human uterus. In the last century it was believed that removing the uterus of a woman prone to 'hysteria' would cure her (hence the name hysterectomy). But as one author satirically observes, true uterine hysteria lies solely with our medical practitioners, and reveals itself differently from country to country:

> In ancient times it [the uterus] used to wander about the body and cause hysteria in the process. At least that is what it was thought to do. Nowadays and thanks to medical knowledge, it is fixed to its ligaments, but this has by no means bridled its erratic behaviour. If only ancient writers had considered that uteri do not wander within bodies but among countries and continents, the term hysteria would have been more aptly derived than it is now.
>
> The larger the uterus, the greater is the hysteria that it can inflict upon its surroundings. Thus if a pregnant uterus wanders into France, it becomes so hyperactive that there is a more than 40 per cent chance that it will need subduing by a range of tocolytic drugs in order to prevent untimely expulsion of the baby. On the other hand, if it wanders into Ireland, it becomes so sluggish that no tocolytic agents are marketed in that country and the odds are two to three that it will need to be driven on by oxytocin to expel a baby that would have fallen out a long time ago, if only it had stayed in France. If it crosses the Atlantic, the chances are that neither of these attempts to curb erratic uterine behaviour will be effective and that one uterus in five will need a scalpel to bring it to its senses and release its contents.[1]

In truth, every uterus behaves a little differently in labour. Labour does not progress like clockwork. Contraction of the uterus and the expansion of the cervix do not always happen at the same time. The levels of pain which a mother feels cannot be predicted. The sooner medical men and women accept these facts, the sooner we can begin to have truly healthier babies and mothers.

Birth is an essentially violent act in the sense that it involves enormous physical force. Ina May Gaskin describes a labouring woman as '... an elemental force – like a tornado, a volcano, an earthquake, or a hurricane, with its own laws of behaviour' and the force of labour as 'older and smarter than you, [something] that always gets what it wants'.[2] Birth technology replaces this natural, even tolerable 'violence' and stress with a premeditated, technologically motivated violence. Today the technological model of violence is considered to be superior to the natural one because of its predictability and because of its alleged scientific basis. But the technological model of birth fails women dismally in the way it puts the doctor instead of the mother and baby in the central, crucial role of the birth drama.

There is no doubt that some of the technology and drugs which are used in modern obstetrics have their place. Under some circumstances they can be life-savers. But far too many women are being told that their lives are being saved when this is not, in fact, the case. Women don't need to be saved from childbirth. They need to feel confident and supported enough to be consumed by it.

Birth is a shocking, enthralling, unique experience, and the ways in which a woman is helped to deal with it often depends on her choice of birth attendant. In her description of childbirth, Suzanne Arms puts it this way:

> At this point the woman, nearly sapped of energy, must rally her reserves to begin pushing the baby out, yet she is now confronted with contractions even more violent than before, coming so hard and fast that they seem to meld together in successive waves, culminating in a shattering explosion that overwhelms her entire body ...
>
> Suddenly nauseous and chilled to the bone, the woman turns to the nearest figure of authority with beseeching eyes and a look on her face that no one who has ever attended a delivery will forget. It is a look of shock and disbelief, a statement all of its own that woman is never so completely and totally alone than at this moment. A beseechingly, pleading, imploring cry for help is often articulated as 'Do Something!', 'I can't go on!', 'Help me!' or words of similar

dramatic power. The response of early Christian man might have been to read his wife the passages from the Scriptures telling her it was her lot to suffer so; the response of modern doctors is to inject drugs to end the suffering. Yet neither reaction is responsible. When primitive woman turned to the midwife with that same look of desperation, the midwife rightfully interpreted the plea to mean 'Assist me', 'Support me', 'Tell me this is supposed to happen.' The obstetrician reads it as a cry to 'Stop it', 'Intervene', 'Do it for me.'[3]

The Active Birth movement, founded by Janet Balaskas in 1969, came about in response to active management and the technological and pharmacological interventions which were threatening to take the birth process completely away from women and their bodies. With active birth, women are encouraged to work with their bodies, and with gravity. They are encouraged to understand the way their bodies function, what part the pelvis, the uterus, the cervix and the baby play in the process of birth. Unlike so many other types of ante-natal preparation, the mother is encouraged to give herself the power and permission to be led by her inclinations instead of fighting them.

When reviewing the methods in this chapter for speeding up labour, relieving the pain of labour and assisting labour, please bear in mind that 'failure to progress' is (next to a previous caesarean) the single biggest reason for a programme of active management. But 'failure to progress' is not a diagnosis. It is simply a subjective point of view based more often on rigid adherence to false timetables (known as partograms or cervicograms) than on sound clinical judgement.

Speeding Labour Up

It's natural for a mother to hope that labour won't last too long. She may be motivated by a desire to see her baby after months of waiting, or perhaps she believes that a short, sharp labour would be better than a long, drawn-out one. However, hoping and/or idly musing about something and actively pursuing it are two different things. Medical practitioners often confuse the two, believing that all women have a profound need to 'get it over with' as soon as possible. Yet many women rightly see induction as interference with a natural process – this is one of the reasons why they write 'birth plans'. An NCT survey reported that the length of labour is, ultimately, unimportant to women provided they have good emotional support, have remained in control and maintained their ability to cope with contractions.[4]

There is almost no good reason to induce or accelerate labour. Yet it is now so common that it is considered a valid, if not vital, part of the process. So much so that there are no accurate figures on how often it is used. It is estimated that in the UK 20 per cent of labours are induced with syntocinon.[5] There appear to be no figures to show how often other methods are used, although individual hospitals can have ARM (artificial rupture of membranes) rates as high as 90 per cent. These practices continue even though it is known that perinatal mortality is not reduced by induction rates of more than 8 to 9.5 per cent.[6] One report concluded that:

> Induced labour is longer and associated with more instrumental deliveries, an increased risk of post-partum haemorrhage and perhaps more importantly, a higher incidence of lower APGAR scores than spontaneous labour. If the point of inducing labour is to reduce risks to the neonate, then it may be failing.[7]

Induction and acceleration are usually only carried out, and considered 'necessary', in hospitals. The reasons why they are considered 'necessary' are often fairly suspect. Some clinicians have attempted to argue that the use of ARM and syntocinon to augment labour is the best way to ensure that women give birth during their attendant's shift at the hospital, thus satisfying women's desire for continuity of care.[8] This is the kind of convoluted reasoning which makes campaigners for woman-centred care weep in despair.

When labour is induced and actively managed, control passes away from the mother and into the hands of medical staff. If she feels that the induction was not necessary or she was not consulted or was pressurized into agreeing to it, she may feel resentful, angry, and violated.

Among the most common reasons for induction or acceleration are:

> going more than two weeks past your EDD
> assumed placental inefficiency
> intrauterine growth retardation
> 'failure to progress'.

Comparison of induced and spontaneous post-mature labours has led to the conclusion that a pregnancy after 42 weeks 'may *affect* perinatal outcome but induction of labour does not *improve* this and that uncomplicated post-maturity is not an indication for induction of labour [my italics]'.[9] Nearly a quarter of neonatal deaths in post-term pregnancies are due to congenital abnormalities (resulting in an over-estimation of the risks of a mother going past her EDD). Research suggests that up to 500 inductions would have to be performed to prevent just one death from post-maturity.[10]

Another condition that doctors worry about is placental inefficiency (where the placenta is no longer providing all the oxygen and nutrients needed to sustain the baby). It is not uncommon for a mother who has gone past her due date to be told that her placenta is no longer functioning and that she is endangering her baby's health. While it is true that there is a point past which the placenta become inefficient, it is impossible to diagnose this by looking at a calendar. Induction poses its own threats to a baby's health, so if you are happy to give your baby a bit more time to put in an appearance, let nature take its course.

Equally, there has not yet been a reliable method developed for identifying growth-retarded babies, and induction of labour seems to have resulted in the birth of many premature, but not growth-retarded, infants. Equally, it has been demonstrated that truly growth-retarded babies do not fare any better for having been delivered early.[11] Should the baby turn out to be premature instead of growth retarded, the increased strength of contractions after an induction may end up doing more harm than good, increasing the likelihood of hypoxia (lack of oxygen) in labour and, in rare cases, of asphyxia (suffocation).

A pause in labour is not a good reason to use hormonal acceleration. Some labours, particularly first labours, simply are long. Often the mother's 'failure to progress' is really the practitioner's 'failure to wait'.[12] With first-time mothers the cervix is less likely to have the elasticity of one which has given birth many times, and also the mother herself may be, unconsciously, more reluctant to go headlong into something of which she has no experience.

It is perfectly normal for there to be periods of activity and rest in labour. Most women with long labours welcome the periods of rest, which give them time to build up their strength and channel their inner resources for the next contraction. If your labour slows down it may be a signal that you need a break and, provided that there is no sign of distress in the baby and you are well, there is no harm in waiting. While you are resting the midwife can continue to check the baby's heartbeat regularly.

The idea of accelerating labour is the cornerstone of active management. In spite of the lack of evidence pointing to the benefits of active management,[13] nearly 40 per cent of the hospitals in one comprehensive survey of all the consultant maternity units in England said that they had a policy for the routine rupture of membranes; of these, the majority (82 per cent) specified that this should be done when the woman is between 2 and 5 cm dilated. Having achieved full dilation, more than half the units (55 per cent) said that they had an upper limit of one hour for the second stage of labour for first-time mothers and half an hour for women having their second or subsequent child. After this time some action would be taken to deliver the baby either instrumentally or surgically.[14]

Doctors are not always able to agree whether slow progress, known as dystocia, is caused by ineffective contractions or an inelastic cervix. This may account for the high failure rates of different types of induction procedures, as there is a certain amount of trial and error involved in deciding whether a woman 'needs' her contractions strengthened or her cervix softened. Between a third and one half of women whose progress is judged to be going too slowly have contractions which are adequate to stretch open the cervix, pointing to some kind of cervical resistance. Half of women judged to have slow labours will progress equally well with or without drugs to 'help' them.[15] Given these facts, it seems the debate over how to make the uterus perform to a particular standard is, in the end, academic.

For women who wish to induce the onset of labour or speed it up there are options which are less invasive, perhaps easier to control, and likely to result in a better outcome and experience of labour for them and their baby. First, if you feel that your labour is overdue but there is no urgent need to have the baby born, try all natural methods first. Nipple stimulation, homoeopathic remedies, lovemaking, eating spicy food, acupuncture, or using a bath or water pool (if available) can help, though not all of these are encouraged in a hospital environment. There is ample evidence to show that simply walking around – occasionally difficult to achieve in hospital – produces as good, if not better, results than any available drugs. If your contractions are not efficient, squatting can make them stronger – so much so that women in established labour may find it painful to get into or maintain the squatting position. Use a stool to help support yourself if you can.

The order in which you should try more drastic measures is a matter of debate among professionals, but the most 'mother-friendly' route (after a dose of caster oil) is considered to be prostaglandin pessaries or gel first, then syntocinon, then ARM (many hospitals start with ARM). That way at least your baby still has the amniotic fluid to protect its head from the powerful contractions which follow an induction.

Managing Labour

ARM – Artificial Rupture of Membranes

The amniotic sac is what protects the baby as it grows, and what cushions it during labour. In some 12 per cent of cases the membranes which contain the amniotic fluid rupture spontaneously at the onset of labour. Otherwise they may rupture of their own accord sometime before or during the second stage.

ARM, also known as amniotomy or 'breaking the waters', is still one of the most common procedures carried out routinely in hospitals across the UK, and can be one of the most potent ways of establishing labour within a few hours. There was a time when it was carried out routinely on every woman on her admission to hospital.

Apart from inducing labour, one of the most common reasons for rupturing the membranes is to check for signs of meconium (faecal material). It is thought that if the baby excretes meconium it is a sign of distress. But on its own meconium staining cannot be considered conclusive evidence of distress, although a combination of staining accompanied by a poor EFM (electronic fetal monitor) reading and a change in the acid-base balance in the baby's blood would give cause for concern.

ARM is an uncomfortable procedure (though it should not be painful). It is usually more successful on women who have had one or more children and/or whose cervix is very 'ripe'. Most practitioners would consider this a simple procedure: an amniohook, not unlike a crochet hook, is pushed up into the cervix until it bursts the bag of amniotic fluid which surrounds the baby. This in turn triggers the release of the natural hormone, prostaglandin, which in turn stimulates the uterus to begin contracting. It is often the first stop on the runaway train of interventions in labour. Even if it is hospital policy, you have a right to refuse ARM if suggested. It should never be done without your knowledge or consent.

Advantages:

* There are no advantages to the routine induction of labour by ARM – when induction is justified, there are usually other less heavy-handed methods that should be tried first.

* If labour is already established and the mother is exhausted, her strength and patience running out, ARM may be justified.

Disadvantages:

* ARM is an invasive and uncomfortable procedure.

* It increases the risk of infection, initially to the mother and later to the baby. While the amniotic sac is intact the baby is in a sterile environment. Once broken, the risk of infection, particularly in hospitals, is increased. If infection sets in, a caesarean will be done.

* The outcome is not guaranteed. Sometimes ARM does not help to establish labour. If this is the case, further interventions will be used. Because of this, ARM is often used in conjunction with a syntocinon drip, resulting in further side-effects for mother and baby.

* ARM can stimulate unnaturally strong contractions which the mother may find difficult to cope with. This can lead to the use of pain-relieving drugs, which also have side-effects.

* After amniotomy, the forewaters, which would normally cushion the baby's head against the force of the contractions, are gone. The baby's head may press against the umbilical cord, sometimes with enough force to crush it. It can also increase the likelihood of excessive moulding

of the baby's head during delivery, making it appear misshapen and, in some cases, causing nerve damage.

✳ Babies born to mothers who have ARM are more likely to have breathing difficulties.

Artificial Hormones
There are two types of artificial hormones used to stimulate labour: synthetic prostaglandin, and syntocinon.

The lining of the uterus contains natural prostaglandin, which is known to play a part in the normal physiology of labour. Because of this the invention of *synthetic prostaglandin* represents something of a breakthrough in induction techniques. Given in the form of pessaries, gel or cream, it gives mothers and doctors a less invasive form of induction which does not restrict a mother's ability to move around. It is not, however, without its side-effects.

The pessaries are usually inserted into the vagina at regular intervals of between 6 and 12 hours. These ripen (soften) the cervix, usually within 24 to 48 hours, which in turn stimulates labour. In most cases labour begins after one or two doses, but if the cervix is very unripe there is quite a high failure rate (around 60 per cent). This can result in women being administered more doses over a longer period of time to try and achieve the same results. However, if the cervix is very unripe it could be because your baby is not ready to be born yet; this gives rise to the question of why anybody would want to force open a cervix which is not ready to give birth. Once the process is begun, though, practitioners will usually want to keep it going. So, if prostaglandin pessaries don't work, you will be put on a syntocinon drip. If this is not successful the next step is a forceps delivery or a caesarean.

Every woman reacts differently to prostaglandin. Some react quickly with powerful contractions – which is why prostaglandin pessaries should not be used on a woman who is already in established labour. While there is some likelihood of an over-stimulated uterus, this is less common than when syntocinon is used. Women who have had a previous caesarean section and who now wish to have a vaginal birth should never be given prostaglandin pessaries, as they soften not just the cervix but the entire uterus, increasing the likelihood of scar rupture.

Syntocinon is a powerful synthetic hormone which is similar to the natural oxytocin produced by the pituitary glands of both mother and baby during labour. It can be used to induce or accelerate labour. It is usually given via an intravenous drip or infusion. This will restrict a woman's ability to move around. Syntocinon usually works immediately, producing incredibly powerful and painful contractions which are longer in duration with shorter gaps in between than non-induced contractions. The drip, once started, will be kept up throughout labour and well after the birth to ensure the delivery of the placenta (at which time the mother will be given a shot of another drug, ergometrine, to counteract the effects of syntocinon and close off the blood vessels in the uterus).

Again, one of the major drawbacks of this method is the powerful contractions which it generates. In a normal labour the intensity of the contractions builds gradually and is met by the body's release of natural pain-killers called endorphins. The syntocinon drip does away with this gradual build-up, eliminating any possibility of the body responding effectively. In the face of overwhelming pain, which can come on quite quickly, the body cannot produce endorphins fast enough to help the mother cope. This is usually when pain-relieving drugs are suggested, and accepted.

In addition, the contractions in a normal labour are shorter, with longer periods of rest in between. During a contraction the blood vessels carrying blood and oxygen to the placenta are temporarily constricted. The placenta deals with this by storing up blood in between contractions to keep a constant supply going to the baby. The greater intensity of the contractions produced by syntocinon means that the baby goes without oxygen for longer than may be safe, increasing the risk of fetal distress.

One Irish study discovered that syntocinon, when used in conjunction with epidural anaesthesia, was likely to increase the probability of scar rupture in women who wished to have a vaginal birth after a previous caesarean.[16] Syntocinon is also associated with a significant degree of water retention in mothers, and neonatal jaundice in babies. Given all this it is probably fair to say that if syntocinon had been invented today instead of in the 1950s, its widespread routine use could not have been justified without further data from clinical trials.

Many women are not aware that if they have a syntocinon drip and are finding the intensity of the contractions too hard to cope with, they can request that the doctor or midwife adjust the speed of the drip. If you want to be mobile, you can request a mobile drip – though these are not always available.

You can greatly help yourself with the pain of induced or accelerated contractions by not lying on your back. If possible a kneeling position, with you leaning forward on a chair, a bed or over a bean bag, is best. When you are lying down the weight of the baby and of your uterus constricts the flow of blood via the main maternal blood vessels, depriving your baby of even more oxygen.

Many practitioners do not like to have women in the kneeling position because they say it interferes with monitoring. This is not usually true, though electronic monitors can be unbelievably fussy and delicate. Monitoring can be done just as easily with the mother in the kneeling position as with the mother in the semi-reclining position. If you find the belt monitor uncomfortable you can request that the midwife uses frequent sonic aid monitoring or Pinard instead.

If you accept induction then another intervention, continuous monitoring, must also be used to detect signs of fetal distress caused by the syntocinon. Like prostaglandin, syntocinon is not 100 per cent successful, so it is often used in conjunction with ARM. However, there is still a failure rate of between 10 and 30 per cent.[17] In these cases a caesarean will be performed. If your practitioner suggests the use of either prostaglandin or syntocinon, he or she should have a convincing reason for doing so. You have the right to refuse any form of induction or acceleration regardless of what stage of labour you are in and whether or not it is 'hospital policy'.

Advantages:

* There are no medical advantages of using prostaglandins or syntocinon to induce or accelerate labour of a normal woman with a healthy baby.

* Some mothers with babies who have died *in utero* may prefer a swift induction rather than waiting for labour to start spontaneously.

Disadvantages:

* The use of synthetic hormones results in the body being unable to produce endorphins, the body's own natural pain-killers, fast enough to help a woman cope with pain naturally.

* The intensity and duration of contractions will be greater, and periods of rest will be shorter. This can be overwhelming and exhausting for the mother and can reduce the amount of oxygen available to the baby, increasing the risk of fetal distress.

* A mother's mobility will be restricted by the use of a drip as well as by the use of the fetal monitor, which must be used when labour is induced.

* Because of the relatively high failure rate of synthetic hormones, there is an increased risk that the labour will end in a caesarean section.

* There is a risk of over-stimulation of the uterus. When this happens uterine activity becomes uncoordinated and the cervix fails to dilate. In the most extreme cases the muscle may go into spasm, causing fetal distress and, very rarely, uterine rupture in an otherwise healthy, unscarred uterus.

* In large doses, syntocinon may cause oedema and high blood pressure.

* Prostaglandin can irritate the smooth muscle of the bowel, causing vomiting, diarrhoea or migraine. It can also cause vaginal irritation or an allergic reaction.

* The risk of post-partum haemorrhage is increased. Large doses of synthetic hormones to induce labour disable the body's ability to close the blood vessels in the womb and expel the placenta. For this reason another drug, ergometrine, will be used.

* Breathing difficulties are most common among babies whose mothers have had their labours induced, especially if the baby is premature. Prematurity is another common result of induction – especially if the dates are wrong. A baby born prematurely will have immature lungs which are not yet ready to function.

* Syntocinon has been linked to an increased risk of jaundice in babies.

Sweeping the Membranes
Although a relatively invasive procedure, sweeping the membranes, which has been practised for more than 100 years, is quite effective and has only one potentially harmful consequence: the accidental (and sometimes deliberate) breaking of a woman's waters. The cervix is covered with a thin membrane which normally stretches apart as the cervix opens up. To dislodge this

membrane your practitioner will usually insert a gloved finger into your vagina, as if he or she were doing an internal examination, and run a finger over the cervix. It can be very painful and it can sometimes cause your membranes to rupture. As it is to the baby's advantage to keep the membranes intact for as long as possible, you should weigh the pros and cons of this procedure up carefully.

To date, the largest randomized, controlled trial to assess the efficacy of sweeping the membranes in post-term pregnancies found that this procedure reduced the duration of pregnancy by between 2 and 5 days.[18] On average 65 per cent of women who had their membranes swept went into labour within three days. The rates of induction were lower in the group of women who had their membranes swept (8 per cent) than for those who did not (19 per cent). Sweeping the membranes is most effective on women whose cervix is already very 'ripe', so it could be argued that it is, ultimately, of little benefit.

There have been no trials to assess the effect which sweeping the membranes has on the mode of delivery or perinatal outcome. However, if you feel you are genuinely 'overdue', asking for this procedure may be a safer alternative for both you and your baby than ARM or hormonal induction. Sometimes practitioners perform this procedure without telling a woman. For instance, a midwife may say she is going to check your dilation and then sweep your membranes. This is an assault. You have the right to be consulted and a right to refuse. Unfortunately, it can be hard, after the fact, to prove that this procedure has been carried out.

Advantages:

* This is a simple procedure which can be done quickly and has few known side-effects.

* For the majority of women who are overdue and/or have a very ripe cervix it can stimulate labour to begin, within an average of three days.

* With this form of induction, your contractions will be of normal intensity and probably more manageable.

* Sweeping the membranes does not upset the delicate hormonal balance of your body and so there is less risk of post-partum haemorrhage.

Disadvantages:

* It is an invasive procedure. Women who are unhappy about internal examinations may not like having their membranes swept.

* It can be very painful.

* Accidental rupture of the membranes is possible. Equally, some practitioners use this procedure deliberately to break a woman's waters.

* It is not very effective for women who do not have a ripe cervix.

* There is an increased risk of infection to the mother and baby.

Monitoring

Monitoring is used to assess the condition of the baby during labour. While technically advanced and impressive-looking machines such as the electronic fetal monitor give us some indication of how the baby, or rather the baby's heartbeat, responds to labour, it fails, for the most part, to do what it sets out to do – namely to detect babies who are at risk in the womb with a view to delivering these babies safely. Because the mother's and the baby's heartbeats vary naturally at different times during labour, it is up to the practitioner to determine when these variations mean trouble.

Nobody would deny the importance of periodic checks on the baby's heartbeat during labour. It is the best possible way for everyone to assure themselves of the baby's continued well-being. Should the rhythm of your baby's heartbeat change significantly, this is a possible indication of fetal distress and may mean that your baby needs some help in being born.

Your baby's heartbeat will normally slow down during a contraction. This is due to the squeezing action of the uterine muscles on the main blood vessels leading, via the placenta, to the baby. The temporary squeezing motion decreases the supply of oxygen to the baby for the duration of the contraction. This is a normal part of the process of labour and will not harm your baby. In circumstances where there have been no interventions, it is usual to employ intermittent monitoring directly after a contraction, usually once an hour. Sometimes the frequency of intermittent monitoring is increased during the second stage of labour, if necessary.

Continuous monitoring is only necessary when there have been interventions or if there is something wrong with your baby. Because many of the interventions used in labour have a direct effect on your baby – either because they are drugs which cross the placenta (epidural anaesthesia, pethidine, Entenox) and alter the baby's heartbeat or because the labour has been artificially accelerated via ARM, syntocinon or prostaglandin – it is usual to have this form of monitoring when in hospital. Much of the distress which is detected in babies is thought to be the direct result of these interventions.

An analysis of several randomized, controlled trials comparing electronic fetal monitoring with intermittent monitoring concluded, 'Sadly, clinicians appear to be more interested in justifying and continuing their own policies than using science to help them formulate safer, more effective policies for monitoring the fetus.'[19] These policies are influenced by the fact that machines are perceived as being more cost-effective than midwives, and that they are more convenient because they do practitioners' thinking for them. In addition, should a parent choose

Managing Labour

to pursue a malpractice claim the fact that the machine was turned on can be held up as an example of good medical 'care'.

Ultimately the diagnosis of fetal distress rests in the hands of whoever is interpreting the data (either by actually listening to the baby's heartbeat or checking the electronic read-outs). If you disagree with the practitioner's interpretation you have the right to ask for another reading or a second opinion. If you disagree with any proposed course of action based on 'fetal distress', you can refuse it.

Depending on the type of monitoring you agree to, you can still maintain freedom of movement during labour. As a rule, continuous fetal monitoring requires that you lie on your back. The belts which are strapped round your middle and the electrodes which are screwed into your baby's scalp can easily become detached, so practitioners will usually want you to stay as still as possible.

A review of studies of various methods of fetal monitoring show that the type of monitoring used is often less important to women than the support they receive from staff and companions.[20] Nevertheless, you should ask questions. Find out what kind of monitoring is most commonly used in the hospital and/or by the practitioner who will be assisting you in labour. Ask how each type might restrict your freedom of movement, both in theory and in practice. Ultimately, you have the right to refuse any form of monitoring during labour if you wish.

Intermittent Monitoring

With intermittent monitoring your baby's heartbeat can be assessed while you are in almost any position – kneeling on all fours, standing, sitting upright, lying down – and can even be done under water in any of these positions. Breathing and relaxing while you are being monitored will help to provide a more accurate reading.

This is the type of monitoring which is most appropriate for normal, uncomplicated labours. It is done every so often instead of continuously, thereby reducing the number of restrictions on a mother during labour and also avoiding the stress of continuously looking for something wrong which continuous monitoring imposes on both mother and practitioner.

There are three types of intermittent monitoring which are currently used: the Pinard (ear trumpet), stethoscope, and Doppler (sonic aid).

Pinard or Ear Trumpet

This simple instrument has a long history in childbirth. When one end is pressed firmly onto your abdomen the midwife can listen to the baby's heartbeat through the other end. She then counts the number of heartbeats per minute – usually by listening for 20 seconds and multiplying the number of beats heard by three. This is an accurate and completely harmless way of assessing your baby's welfare.

Stethoscope

An ordinary doctor's stethoscope can be used in exactly the same way as a Pinard, with the same results. Some midwives find it easier to use when the woman is in an upright position. The stethoscope can also be handed to the woman so she can have the opportunity of hearing her baby's heartbeat for herself.

Doppler or Sonic Aid

The Doppler or sonic aid is an ultrasonic device (a fact which is seldom explained to mothers); any mother who wishes to avoid exposing her baby to ultrasound should be cautious of the overuse of what appears to be a harmless little gadget. With the sonic aid, small quantities of ultrasound waves are used to magnify the sound of the baby's heartbeat. Doppler ultrasound is used mainly to detect the flow of blood and this is what you hear, interpreted as a heartbeat. This machine has the advantage that both the mother and the practitioner can hear the heartbeat, which many mothers find reassuring.

Sonic aids come in all shapes and sizes. There are small portable versions which can be used in the home, and there are larger ones which are used in hospitals and which can also produce a graphic printout of the rhythm of your baby's heartbeat. Dopplers can even be used underwater, in which case a transducer (a small patch with a wire which is attached to the machine) is pressed against the mother's abdomen near the spot where the baby's heart lies.

Advantages:

* Intermittent monitoring decreases the likelihood of the baby being wrongly diagnosed as 'in distress'.

* It is less invasive than continuous monitoring.

* It can be done with the mother in any position, and even under water.

* It increases the amount of personal attention a mother gets from her attendants and encourages practitioners to use their clinical judgement instead of letting machines do their thinking for them.

Disadvantages:

* Provided both mother and baby are healthy, there are no disadvantages to intermittent monitoring.

* Dopplers and sonic aids are ultrasonic devices. Mothers who are concerned about unnecessary exposure should avoid them if possible.

Continuous Monitoring
This form of monitoring is most appropriately applied when there have been interventions in the normal process of labour. Fetal monitoring has become such a part of the routine of labour in UK hospitals that very few stop to question its validity.

When a woman first enters hospital she is likely to be told she must have a 20- or 30-minute session of *Cardiotocographic Monitoring* (CTG) to provide a baseline reading of her baby's heartbeat. Once you submit to this you will probably be asked to repeat the process every two hours or so. Studies have shown that there are no special advantages to this type of monitoring over the less invasive types. One of the largest trials ever comparing intermittent monitoring with continuous monitoring was conducted in Dublin. It concluded that, with the exception of detecting the possibility of seizures in a small group of high-risk babies whose mothers were in labour for more than five hours or where labour was induced, there was no difference in birth outcome between groups of mothers who were continuously monitored and those who were monitored intermittently.[21] The findings showed that continuous electronic fetal monitoring (EFM) made almost no difference at all in terms of reducing caesarean rates, inductions, instrumental deliveries, or the number of babies who need resuscitation after birth. Nor did it improve stillbirth and neonatal death rates or APGAR scores.

EFMs tend to make practitioners anxious and jumpy. This in turn can affect the way a mother feels about her labour. Some women have reported that the procedure, which involves strapping the mother into an abdominal belt, is disruptive and, because they are usually asked to lie down during this period, uncomfortable. A reading can be taken while you are upright, but a woman who is upright may naturally move around more than one lying down and it is very difficult to get a reliable reading if the woman moves because the monitor may slip and the trace may not be long or clear enough to provide good data.

There are two ways of continuously monitoring a woman and her baby in labour: with an abdominal belt monitor and with scalp electrodes.

Abdominal Belt Monitor
A belt or an elastic band is sited around the mother's abdomen to hold the transducer, which is an ultrasonic device, in place.

Sometimes there are two transducers – one to measure the rhythm of the baby's heartbeat and the other to measure the strength of the contractions. The resulting printout is a continuous graph which reflects the baby's heartbeat in relation to the mother's contractions.

Advantages:

* Provided the machine is in good working order, this kind of monitoring can be very reassuring if interventions are being used or if the baby is at risk.

Disadvantages:

* If the machine cuts out unexpectedly it may cause unnecessary panic about the baby's condition. Furthermore, if the machine breaks down entirely some doctors are not confident enough to carry on with a labour unless another working machine can be found. In these cases a caesarean will be performed.

* There is an increased incidence of caesarean section in mothers who are continuously monitored – even if the machine is working.

* The interpretation of the data depends very much on the condition of the machine, as well as on the subjective attitudes of the practitioner. False readings do occur, and these are a major cause of unnecessary interventions.

* Monitors are often used as a substitute for personal care and, worse, as a substitute for rational thought and skill. Practitioners can fall into the trap of watching the monitor instead of paying attention to the mother.

* Most hospitals insist that a mother who is being monitored should lie down. This increases the likelihood of fetal distress as the weight of the uterus and the baby pressing on the main blood vessels leading to the placenta impair the blood supply, and therefore oxygen supply, to the baby.

* Many women find the CTG belts uncomfortable. This added discomfort can make the pain of contractions even more difficult to bear.

* These machines are quite hypnotic. Watch them for too long and you can begin to believe that it is the machine which is keeping your baby alive instead of yourself. This can sap a mother's confidence.

* The transducers in the CTG belt use ultrasound to detect the baby's heartbeat and the strength of contractions.

Scalp Electrode

If your baby is diagnosed as being at risk, this form of monitoring may be used. To be accurate it should be used in conjunction with fetal blood sampling. An electrode on the end of a spiral or s-shaped hook is screwed into the baby's scalp through the mother's dilating cervix. If the mother's membranes have not already ruptured, then they will be artificially ruptured beforehand. Once the electrode is attached the mother is discouraged from moving around, though some upright positions are possible. This form of monitoring should never be used in a normal labour.

Advantages:

* When used in conjunction with the measurement of fetal blood sampling, this is considered by many practitioners to be the most accurate method of assessing the baby's welfare.

Managing Labour

* It can provide the reassurance that, should the baby's condition truly deteriorate, your practitioner can react swiftly to help your baby be born safely.

Disadvantages:

* Early artificial rupturing of the membranes, which must be done to attach the electrode, increases the risk of infection and increases pressure on the baby's head throughout labour and particularly during the second, 'pushing', stage. It also makes contractions longer, more intense and more painful.

* This is a very invasive form of monitoring.

* There is some evidence that hooking the monitor into the scalp is painful for the baby. Babies who have been subjected to this kind of monitoring often have wounds on their scalps which can leave bald spots on their heads. The open wounds can be sites of serious infections.

* Full mobility for the mother is not possible. Some mobility might be possible, depending on the length of the wire which leads to the main processor and the good will of your attendants.

* In hospitals where this form of monitoring is used routinely in normal labours, the number of caesareans is unusually high, sometimes 25 per cent or more.

* To be really accurate it should be used in conjunction with fetal blood sampling – another invasive procedure – to confirm that the baby is really in distress.

Telemetry

This is a form of monitoring which is similar to the scalp electrode, but which uses radio waves instead of electronic impulses. An electrode transmitter is attached to the baby's head in the same way as the scalp electrode, requiring the rupture of the membranes. But because there is no wire there is greater freedom of movement. Most of the risks which apply to the scalp electrode are relevant to the use of telemetry.

Pain

The fact is that childbirth is painful. Pain is part of the process – so much so that some believe if you take away the pain you take away the experience as well. Certainly the pain of childbirth is one of the reasons why doctors believe it to be a pathological condition. Doctors see part of their duty as relieving human suffering, and if they are dealing with someone with a broken arm or a brain tumour this interpretation may be correct. But the pain of childbirth is not pathological, it is purposeful. In normal, physiological labours it is rarely unmanageable or totally overwhelming provided the woman is upright and has all the support and encouragement she needs.

Because the pain of childbirth is a universal experience, we can assume that it is pain, not painlessness, which is normal. Since nature rarely does anything without a purpose it's worth asking what the purpose of pain in labour might be. The answer seems to be that it's physiological as well as psychological. Physiologically, women need to know when they are in labour. They need to know how far along they are and whether the birth of their baby is imminent. The different types and levels of pain which a woman feels at different stages of labour provide this information.

Psychologically, working with or submitting to the power of labour offers an opportunity for self-discovery which is unique to women. Those who have experienced labour without pain-relieving drugs may go through a powerful psychological transition, which women who have chosen to eliminate the pain may not experience. In the light of this, taking away the pain of childbirth may significantly 'diminish [its] quality and significance'.[22]

Certainly there is no evidence that women's levels of satisfaction with birth are linked to the absence of pain. In fact, the group of women who are most likely to express dissatisfaction with birth are those who have had epidurals and had no sensation of pain at all.[23]

But when all is said and done, pain is usually the one thing (next to tearing or episiotomy) that women fear most. In response to women's cries for help there have been a number of different drugs – analgesics, tranquillizers and anaesthesia – offered to relieve the pain of childbirth. Some are more effective than others and, ironically, the more effective a drug is at relieving the mother's pain, the greater the number of adverse effects it has on her baby.

It's part of the perverse nature of medicine that health practitioners see it as their duty to discourage mothers from smoking or drinking during pregnancy, then, when they go into labour, inject them with some of the most powerful drugs known to man. How can it be that drugs, when taken socially or for pleasure, are 'proven' to have damaging side-effects for mothers and babies, yet those which are administered for alleged medical purposes have none? A drug is a drug is a drug, no matter if it is prescribed in a hospital or bought on a street corner, and all drugs produce side-effects.

In a normal labour the level of pain builds gradually, allowing the body time to respond by releasing endorphins – natural hormonal pain-killers – when the body is pushed beyond its normal limits. Endorphins are similar to opiates and can give relief from pain and produce a dreamlike state in the mother. Endorphin production stops when an epidural is administered, though pethidine and Entenox (gas and air) do not appear to inhibit their production.

All women use pain relief in labour. Their methods can range from self-help techniques such as being upright, being mobile, yoga, meditation, music, massage, homoeopathic remedies and various breathing techniques to less invasive (though often not very effective) paraphernalia such as the TENS machine.

From a medical point of view, however, pain relief falls into two categories: analgesic and anaesthetic. Analgesic pain relief is designed to assist a mother with the normal pains of labour. It is much like the kind of pain relief you would take for a headache – though obviously much stronger. It is a general pain reliever which works on the whole body rather than specifically sited parts. It takes the edge off pain but does not eliminate it. Anaesthetic pain relief is designed to be used selectively to relieve the pain of obstetric interventions and operative procedures. It is usually targeted at a specific place on the body, such as the spine or perineum. Anaesthetics eliminate pain completely.

Levels of pain in labour are not predestined and they can change according to the kind of social support a mother has, whether she feels safe in her place of birth, her own level of fear about the birth process, what position her body is in, the way the baby is lying and what interventions, if any, she has had. There are many methods of natural pain relief available, but for a mother in hospital whose labour is being medically directed these are likely to be pretty ineffective. A woman who wishes to manage labour pains with her own resources might be best advised to do this from the beginning, before any interventions in labour are used. For her, pharmacological methods of pain relief would be considered only as a last resort.

When using drugs in labour it is important to be able to assess the extent to which the cervix has dilated. If the cervix is nearly fully dilated (between 7 and 10 cm), it may be better to avoid some forms of pain relief that can slow down the second stage of labour and cause the baby's condition to deteriorate. Used early on in labour, many of the drugs used for pain relief have had time to be cleared out of the mother's system. When drugs are used during the later stages of labour there is a greater risk that they will remain in the baby's bloodstream after birth and take longer to clear. The baby's fragile system then has to cope with the extra burden of trying to detoxify itself at the same time as it is adjusting to life outside the womb.

You also have the right to know about any side-effects which pain-relieving drugs may have for you or your baby. Unfortunately, some doctors and midwives are terribly misinformed about the efficacy or side-effects of most of the drugs which they use routinely, and this misinformation gets passed on to mothers. The most common misconception is that pain-relieving drugs, especially the epidural, do not cross the placenta. ALL drugs cross the placenta, though some appear to do less damage than others. What you put into your body you put into your baby's body as well.

Often, when considering the use of pain-relieving drugs, we tend to focus on the immediate future both in terms of benefits and side-effects. However, studies of the long-term effects on babies whose mothers used drugs during labour make disturbing reading. These show a link between drug use in labour and drug addiction in later life.[24] This is due to what is known as 'imprinting' – a specific memory engraved during a short, sensitive period – in this case, the crucial hours of labour – leading to specific behaviours in adult life. While addiction itself is not the result of imprinting, the tendency to use and abuse drugs is thought to be. Labour involves a certain amount of stress for both mother and baby. If during this important time drugs which relieve that stress enter the baby's bloodstream, the baby has received an imprinted message that this is the appropriate response to stress. The greater availability and social acceptability of drugs today mean that more and more young adults may respond to this unconscious imprint later in life.

Having said this, labouring without drugs should not be considered a test of womanhood. If you are genuinely experiencing more pain than you can cope with, and if alternative methods have failed to produce the desired relief, you should have access to effective pharmacological pain relief. If you ask for it, it should not be denied to you, nor should you be made to feel as if you have failed because you need it. Equally, if you wish to have a drug-free labour, nobody has the right to force you to accept any drug which you do not want. The choice is entirely yours.

Gas and Air

This method of pain relief, also known as Entenox, is composed of equal proportions of nitrous oxide (laughing gas) and oxygen. To use it the mother places a rubber mask over her mouth at the beginning of a contraction and inhales deeply. The mask is fitted with a valve which opens when she inhales and closes when she exhales. The anaesthetic effect lasts about 60 seconds.

Entenox does not take the pain away, but combined with the slow, deep breaths you will need to take to inhale the mixture, it can help take the edge off. Nobody has compared simple deep breathing with Entenox to assess whether it is the drug or the breathing which is the most effective. Inhaling Entenox can make you feel a bit light-headed, dizzy or nauseous. It clears out of your and your baby's system quickly, if used in moderation, and appears to have little long- or short-term side-effects.

The best time to use gas and air is probably at the end of the first stage during the very strong contractions of transition. However, if you are in great pain, Entenox probably won't help. If used during the second stage of labour, the deep breaths needed to inhale the drug may interfere with the bearing down efforts needed to help expel the baby, and may thus delay the birth.

Because of the nature of the drug it is only useful for a little while. While relatively benign in small doses, over-use of Entenox does alter your state of consciousness and can make you feel nauseous, confused, disorientated and disconnected from the experience of labour.

Pethidine

Pethidine is a powerful narcotic derived from morphine. It is given via an intramuscular injection into the thigh or bottom and acts on the nerve cells in the brain and spinal cord. Rather than taking the pain away, it alters the mother's state of consciousness and therefore her perception of pain. Most women find it a completely ineffective pain reliever. It does, however, seem to be an effective muscle relaxant, so while it may not combat pain it may help cervical dilation if the first stage of labour has been prolonged. However, it can leave women feeling as if they have lost the courage, the inclination and the ability to cope. Because nausea is a common side-effect, pethidine is sometimes given in combination with tranquillizers or mood-altering drugs to stop the mother feeling queasy. The combined effect means that a mother loses the ability and will to give birth herself, increasing the likelihood of other interventions being used. Pethidine in repeated or very high doses can slow down a mother's breathing, thus decreasing the amount of oxygen available to the baby. This can lead to fetal distress.

Pethidine and any tranquillizers used in conjunction with it can cross the placenta and go directly into the baby's system, increasing the possibility that the baby will have breathing difficulties at birth. A significant proportion of babies whose mothers have used pethidine need to be resuscitated and/or given an antidote drug, Naloxone, to bring them round. This effect is more pronounced if the baby is premature or small, particularly if the pethidine is injected very near the time of birth. Babies born to mothers who have used pethidine tend to be drowsy and unresponsive. They may have difficulty suckling which, if prolonged, can cause weight loss. It can take days for the drug to be excreted out of the baby's system, increasing the need for these babies to be assisted with both breathing and feeding. For this reason many paediatricians recommend women use other forms of pain relief. The usual dose has come down in recent years from as much as 200 mg to between 12 and 25 mg because of the adverse effect on the baby. These lower doses render the effects of the drug minimal. It is best taken, without the tranquillizers, before the cervix reaches 7-cm dilation.

Diamorphine
Otherwise known as heroin, this powerful drug is, unbelievably, still being used for pain-relieving purposes in labour in some

parts of the country (particularly the North of England and Scotland). In 1993 a survey revealed that 2.1 per cent of mothers were given heroin in labour.[25] How can this be justified?

The potential side-effects for mother and baby are obvious. Heroin does not take away the pain. Instead it greatly alters a woman's perception of pain and may also make her drowsy. The most immediate physiological side-effect is respiratory depression – mothers with any kind of breathing difficulty should never be given heroin. There will be a drop in blood pressure and body temperature. In some cases the mother will become delirious and suffer allergic reactions (a common response to all opiates). Many midwives and doctors have no idea what a mother's past history of drug use or abuse is. The use of heroin in labour could, inadvertently, send a formerly drug-dependent woman back on the path to addiction.

Babies born to mothers who have used heroin in labour are usually 'flat'. They can be slow to breathe and suck, and generally have low APGAR scores. They may suffer emotional and psychological shock while the drug is clearing from their systems, and so may be more 'fussy' and ill than other babies.

Always find out what's in the syringe before it is injected into you. Mothers tend to report receiving heroin much less often than practitioners report using it.[26] If anyone suggests 'a wee jag' of diamorphine in labour, tell them to get stuffed.

General Anaesthetic
The complete relief from pain which epidurals provide means that there is almost no reason to administer a general anaesthetic to a woman giving birth, save for the most dire emergencies where time is of the essence, such as in the case of an immediate caesarean or, occasionally, the delivery of a second twin. Should a situation arise which calls for an immediate caesarean section, a general anaesthetic can be administered and produce the desired effect of knocking the mother out cold in less than a minute.

The anaesthetic is introduced into the woman's arm via a thin plastic tube. Generally it will take effect within 30 seconds.

While it is taking effect the anaesthetist will put pressure on a specific site on the mother's neck in order to stop the contents of her stomach being regurgitated. Once she is unconscious a tube will be run down her trachea (windpipe) to ventilate her artificially during the operation. There is a rubber cuff around the tube which must be inflated to ensure that vomit does not enter the trachea. Once this is done the anaesthetist releases the pressure on the mother's neck.

However, a general anaesthetic is not without risks. Chief among these is that the mother will regurgitate the contents of her stomach and then inhale them, causing respiratory arrest. This is the fourth most common reason for maternal deaths in the UK. Because of this, doctors say, it is safer to starve women who are in labour in hospitals and dose them up regularly with antacids, keeping both the contents of the stomach and acidity levels to a minimum.

In those rare cases when a woman has become ill or died from the inhalation of her own vomit, it is down to faulty technique on the part of the anaesthetist and support staff, not because the woman has eaten a meal.

The after-effects of a general anaesthetic include nausea, neck and shoulder pain and sore throat as well as confusion, nightmares and hallucinations. Babies born to mothers who have had a general anaesthetic are often 'flat' and can suffer from (occasionally severe) breathing difficulties.

Epidurals
The promise of a completely pain-free birth is a seductive one for many women, and the epidural is the one form of pain relief which lives up to its promise. It is without a doubt the most effective way to eradicate completely any sensations of pain (and any other physical sensations a mother may have) during labour. However, the drug used for epidurals, bupivacaine, is a cocaine derivative, the potential dangers of which are self-evident.

The name epidural is used to describe several different kinds of spinal anaesthesia. A *spinal block* is a single injection of local anaesthetic given between two vertebrae in the lower spine. It is quicker to perform than an epidural, but the effect does not last as long. Some hospitals offer it routinely instead of an epidural for caesareans. Others reserve its use for situations where there is not time to site an epidural and where a general anaesthetic might be inadvisable. Another single injection method is the *pudenal block*, where the anaesthetic is injected inside the vagina to numb the area around the vagina and between the vagina and the anus. This is usually done just before delivery. With the *epidural*, an injection of local anaesthetic is given to numb the lower back. The anaesthetic is then fed continuously via a thin plastic tube (a cannula) into what is known as the epidural space, which lies between the spinal cord and the vertebrae in the spine. Depending on where on the spine the injection is made, a woman can have either total loss of feeling from the breasts down or loss of feeling in the abdomen only. Siting an epidural is an extremely skilled job which must be done by a qualified anaesthetist.

Women may feel frustrated at the lack of information which they get about a procedure which sounds almost too good to be true. They are no more frustrated than those who for the last 30 years have been trying to gather more substantive information about its side-effects. It is estimated that while millions of women all over the world have had epidurals, less than 600 have participated in well-run, controlled trials to assess the possible long-term effects.[27] Furthermore, because so many millions of women have had epidurals it is now difficult (though not impossible) to find a large enough 'control' group of non-epidural women, and babies, to compare them with.

While it is often recommended by doctors as the best possible form of pain relief, many women have found that even if they book an epidural, when they go into hospital there is not one available – usually because chronic understaffing of labour wards means that an anaesthetist cannot be found. These women may end up disappointed by having to wait a long time to have what they wanted or ultimately by not having the pain relief of their choice. In around 8 per cent of cases the epidural drug does not take effect. The reasons for this are not fully understood. I have known women who have been told 'you're resistant to the drug' and even, when the anaesthetist couldn't site the epidural properly, 'you're back is too hard!', though I have yet to hear of an anaesthetist saying 'I did it wrong.'

Be aware that the pain-eradicating effects of an epidural leave it open to a certain amount of abuse by practitioners, who may be tempted to crank up the syntocinon drip and push the uterus to contract harder than ever. This obviously increases the risk of uncoordinated uterine activity, uterine spasm and uterine inefficiency when the time comes to push the baby out, increasing the risk of eventual forceps/ventouse deliveries and caesareans. And all of this without the mother ever knowing what has gone on.

If you elect to have an epidural you will be subjected to a whole range of other procedures. You will need to have electronic fetal monitoring (EFM) because the drug crosses the placenta within minutes of being administered and can affect the baby. While it does not produce the limpness and breathing difficulties which other drugs do, your baby may have decreased muscle tone and strength, be less responsive to the human voice, be more irritable and less able to orientate itself and respond to its surroundings for as long as six weeks after birth.

You will probably have a uterine monitor in conjunction with the EFM to assess the strength of your contractions. Because you will not feel anything, and therefore not cry out, your attendants will have no other way of assessing how far your labour has progressed.

One recently discovered and potentially dangerous side-effect of the epidural is that it can lead to significantly high temperatures in the womb. A baby *in utero* depends entirely on his mother's body for temperature regulation. A woman who has an epidural will herself feel very hot because she is retaining more heat by sweating and breathing less. In an important study comparing epidurals to other forms of pain relief, researchers found that in 30 per cent of babies whose mothers had epidurals, the skin temperature exceeded 38°C (100.4°F); in 10 per cent it exceeded 39°C (102.2°F). The authors of this study found that prolonged use of an epidural can lead to significant hyperthermia (overheating) in the fetus, and that, while no adverse effects were found in the infants in the study, these temperatures were comparable to those which had been shown in previous studies to compromise or damage health in both animals and humans.[28]

Another side-effect of the epidural drug is that it dilates the peripheral blood vessels. Once the drug enters the body there is a noticeable drop in blood pressure (caused by the fact that there is literally not enough liquid to fill up the dilated blood vessels), which can adversely affect the flow of blood and oxygen to the baby. Because of this you will be given an intravenous drip in your arm before the epidural is sited, to keep blood liquid levels up. You will not be able to feel when you need to go to the toilet (and would not be able to walk to the loo anyway). Because of this, you will have a catheter inserted into your urethra which will drain your urine into a plastic bag at the side of your bed.

Because you will not be able to move (unless you have a 'mobile' epidural, which does not totally numb your legs) you might be lying on your back for long periods of time. This has two possibly dangerous side-effects: First, the weight of the baby pressing down on the main maternal blood vessels means that less blood reaches the baby. This can cause fetal distress. Secondly, lying on your back for long periods of time during labour can damage your back. It is unclear, due to lack of research, whether the long-term backache associated with epidurals is because of the drug or because of the position which many women are forced to lie in for extended periods of time, or down to both. If you have an epidural, ask the midwife to help you to lie on your side instead of your back. Your contractions will be more efficient and your baby will fare better. Also, with the help of your birth companions, make sure you change sides from time to time.

Women are often reassured that epidurals are safe for them and for their babies. This has never been proven. But, one study showed that 63 per cent of obstetricians believe that giving a woman an epidural improves their own job satisfaction,[29] which may be one reason why they come so highly recommended! There are, however, a number of chronic side-effects which range from dizziness and tingling hands and fingers to migraines, numbness in the legs and severe backache. Far from being temporary, one study in 1992 which looked back at 11,701 women who had had epidurals at a single hospital in Birmingham between the years of 1978 and 1985 found that about two thirds were still suffering the side-effects of the epidurals which they had had many years before.[30] In the US, where drug manufacturers are obliged to disclose all possible side-effects of drugs on their packaging, the warnings included in the bupivacaine package make enlightening reading (explanations in square brackets are mine):

> Local anaesthetics rapidly cross the placenta, and when used for epidural, caudal or pudenal block anaesthesia, can cause varying degrees of maternal, fetal and neonatal [newborn] toxicity. The incidence and degree of toxicity depend on the procedure performed, the type and amount of the drug used and the technique of the drug administration. Adverse reactions in the parturient [mother], fetus and neonate involve alteration of the central nervous system, peripheral vascular tone and cardiac function ...
>
> Neurological effects following epidural or caudal anaesthesia may include spinal block [paralysis] of varying magnitude (including high or total spinal block); hypotension [lowered blood pressure] secondary to spinal block; urinary retention; faecal and urinary incontinence [loss of bladder and bowel control]; loss of perineal sensation and sexual function; persistent anaesthesia; paresthesia [numbness in lower limbs], weakness, paralysis of the lower extremities and loss of sphincter control [the muscle surrounding the anus], all of which may have slow, incomplete or no recovery; headache, backache, septic meningitis; meningismus; slowing of labour; increased incidence of forceps delivery, cranial nerve palsies [paralysis, often with involuntary

tremors] due to traction on nerves from loss of cerebrospinal fluid [leakage of the fluid which surrounds the brain].[31]

One small, well-conducted study compared two groups of normal first-time mothers in spontaneous labour. One group received epidural analgesia and the other received narcotic analgesia during labour. In the epidural group there was a significant prolonging of the first and second stages of labour and a significant slowing in the rate of cervical dilation. These women in turn required an increased use of drugs to induce and augment labour. Epidural was associated with an increase in malposition of the baby in 19 per cent of cases (as opposed to 4 per cent of the narcotic group), and a caesarean rate which was more than 10 times greater (25 per cent as opposed to 2 per cent).[32]

These last two findings are not surprising, since the epidural is known to cause the pelvic muscles (which would normally help the baby rotate into optimum position to be born) to become limp and ineffective.

So is the new mobile epidural the answer? With it some (though not all) women still have the use of their legs, and can walk around, presumably working with gravity to help the baby be born and reducing the risk of fetal distress and long-term backache. Many are sceptical. A mobile epidural is still an epidural and the drug still crosses the placenta. The fact that the mother can walk may be seen as helpful but sometimes it's downright dangerous. As American childbirth campaigner Doris Haire comments:

> Will the 'walking epidural' be the answer to a safe, painless childbirth experience? Let us not hold our breath in anticipation. Women have fallen while walking with the 'walking epidural'. The problem seems to result from the fact that a woman can not always be sure that her feet are placed in the proper position to sustain her changing gait.[33]

Until the medical establishment begins to look more seriously at the short- and long-term side-effects of the epidural, it is wrong to state that this form of pain relief is completely 'safe and effective'. Women who have epidurals are taking part in one of the biggest unofficial research trials (after ultrasound) today. The possible ramifications of this must be weighed up carefully against the immediate benefits.

Advantages:

✳ The epidural usually completely eliminates all the painful sensations of childbirth.

✳ For caesarean births it allows the mother to remain awake and fully conscious throughout. She will be able to hold and feed her baby very soon after the operation.

✳ If left in, the epidural can provide post-operative pain relief (though leaving it in is unwise, since there are analgesics which are just as effective at relieving post-operative pain and which have fewer side-effects).

✳ A well-timed epidural – not too late in the first stage, with a low dose that can wear off so that sensation returns in time for second stage pushing – means that some women can deliver their babies without further assistance. Some mothers describe this as a very positive experience.

Disadvantages:

✳ Mothers who have an epidural have an increased likelihood of unnecessary forceps, ventouse and caesarean deliveries.

✳ Episiotomy rates are higher for women with epidurals because they have lost the necessary muscle tone to push the baby out, and require instrumental deliveries.

Every Woman's BirthRights

* A mother who has an epidural will almost always have a completely obstetrically-directed birth, whether she wanted one or not.

* Epidural headache is common when the dura – the protective coating around the spinal chord – is accidentally punctured resulting in fluid from the spinal column leaking into the dural space. This in turn reduces the amount of fluid which the brain floats in, causing severe headaches.

* Backache is one of the many long-term side-effects of epidural, though whether caused by the drug or the fact that the mother has to lie on her back for extended periods of time, is unclear.

* Paralysis can last long after the drug leaves the mother's system. Even when it goes away, some women report tingling in the hands and legs for a long time afterwards.

* Bupivacaine crosses the placenta and can have an adverse effect on the baby's health. Baby's born to mothers who have had epidurals tend to be less alert and often have difficulty breathing and suckling.

* Some babies are born with a slight blue tint – due to imperfect oxygenation of the mother's blood.

* Side-effects for the baby can last for anywhere from 48 hours to six weeks. Mothers who have 'fussy' babies after having an epidural may need to exercise greater patience while the baby suffers the inevitable side-effects of clearing a powerful drug out of its system.

Assisting Labour

When labour is progressing normally and both mother and baby are healthy there is hardly ever any need to assist the birth of the baby. Sometimes women and their practitioners panic at the 'pushing' stage of labour and try to get it over with as quickly as possible. At other times, a woman who has been given drugs to speed up her labour may be so exhausted by the time it comes to give birth that she simply has no strength to push. Either that or her uterus will be so over-stimulated that these final, crucial contractions are beyond its capabilities. In these circumstances practitioners will perform episiotomies, use forceps or vacuum extraction or, in an increasing number of cases, perform a caesarean section.

Episiotomy
With the exception of cutting the umbilical cord, episiotomy is the most common surgical procedure performed on women today.[34] What's more, it is one that is often done without ever consulting the mother.

When a woman in labour is free to assume any position in which she feels comfortable and confident, especially if she maintains an upright position while giving birth, an episiotomy is hardly ever necessary. Rates of episiotomy vary from hospital to hospital and from consultant to consultant in the same hospital, but on the whole there is no excuse for any hospital or practitioner to have an episiotomy rate of over 10 per cent. Amazingly, in the UK the rate of episiotomy is not even officially recorded, but best estimates put the level at between 50 and 90 per cent.[35] Most of these are on first-time mothers. Although episiotomy has been used for centuries, it is only recently that it has reached the vast proportions we see today.

The rationale behind episiotomy is that it eases delivery by making the opening which the baby's head and body pass through bigger. Most episiotomies are right medio-lateral cuts (a sideways cut directed towards the right of the vaginal opening).

This type of cut, preferred in the UK (in the US the midline cut which extends from the vagina to just short of the anus is more prevalent), runs between muscles instead of cutting through them and is done (as far as is possible) away from large blood vessels and nerves. Some practitioners feel that the straight line of the episiotomy is easier to repair and will heal better than if one were not done and the woman were to suffer a tear instead. This of course depends on the kind of tear they are talking about. When birth happens with the woman in an upright position there is usually no tearing and, if there is, it is usually minimal (first-degree, involving skin and fascia only, or small second-degree, involving skin and muscle) and requires no stitching. Giving birth in a semi-recumbent position means giving birth against gravity, and this may result in more serious tears, in which case an episiotomy may be preferable.

Many women do not trust the physiological fact that their bodies will stretch open to assist the birth of their babies. They are terribly frightened of the idea that their bodies might tear or burst open during labour. This fear is often exploited by practitioners, who are maybe in a hurry or who may themselves not trust the process. The women who are most likely to tear are the ones who are being urged to push vigorously during the second stage of labour. There is something to be said for the idea that the word 'push' should be banned from every delivery room in the country, because it encourages women to force a process which normally their bodies can complete quite well in their own good time. Women also tear because some midwives actively manage this stage by forcing the perineum over the baby's head as it is crowning.

If you are having a forceps delivery then you will automatically be given an episiotomy to make room for the forceps to be inserted into your vagina. Some practitioners argue that, in cases of premature birth, episiotomy should be used to protect the baby's head from unnecessary trauma while being forced against the perineal muscle. But, provided there has been no ARM (artificial rupture of the membranes) or other form of augmentation which increases the force of contractions, there is little evidence to support this. Some practitioners still believe that episiotomy reduces the incidence of vaginal prolapse (where the muscles and ligaments which support the vagina become weak, causing it to protrude out of the body). While vaginal prolapse has become more rare in the last 40 years, there is no evidence to show that episiotomy is the reason for this.[36]

Much depends on the timing of the episiotomy as well. An episiotomy performed too early, when the perineum has not thinned out to its fullest extent, will cut not only skin but muscle tissue as well. This will be more difficult to repair and take longer to heal.

In some cases it is not the cut but the repair which is the real problem. Many practitioners, doctors and midwives alike, are unskilled at sewing up perineums. Indeed, it's still common in some areas for students to 'practise' their suturing technique on this delicate part of a woman's anatomy. The reasoning behind this is that the perineum is not a vital organ and so it won't matter much if they make mistakes. You can insist that a qualified practitioner, not a student, repairs the cut.

In addition, the perineum *does* in fact guard the entrance to a vital organ. It is the first point of contact in sexual intercourse, and will stretch over the head of a woman's next baby should she choose to give birth again. The botched jobs sometimes done on women's perineums never used to be so obvious. But as oral sex among adults is more commonplace today, women's genitals are increasingly more on show to their partners, heightening women's self-consciousness and feelings of having been mutilated. Because the trauma of episiotomy occurs in a very private place, many women don't like to talk about it even to their doctors. Instead they suffer silently, unable to stand or sit in one position for long periods of time, unable to enjoy sexual intercourse, and in constant pain. A badly stitched-up perineum is not only ugly and uncomfortable, it can effectively put an end to a woman's sex life. Penetration may be painful, not just for weeks but for years afterwards. Those women who do complain are sometimes offered operations to repair the area. This involves more cutting and stitching, and often second (and in some cases many subsequent) operations only compound the misery of the first.

One way to avoid this is to insist that no episiotomy is to be performed on you routinely and that, if episiotomy is suggested, you get a full explanation of why it is necessary. Many practitioners use the excuse that there isn't time to seek the woman's permission or to give her an explanation, and that in most instances the woman is so far into labour that she cannot be relied upon to make a reasonable judgement (i.e. agree with them). Some are in such a hurry that they don't even wait for the anaesthetic to take effect, or simply don't give an anaesthetic because they believe (wrongly) that there is no feeling in the vaginal tissues after delivery. Don't allow anyone to stitch you up before you have been properly anaesthetized. For all these reasons it is important that you have a partner with you who is there to protect your rights, who understands what you want and, if necessary, can articulate this to your carers.

Advantages:

* There are no proven medical advantages to routine episiotomy.

* Can help with a rapid delivery in an emergency or if the baby is in trouble.

* Episiotomy can facilitate a forceps delivery, limiting the damage to a mother's internal organs caused by the forceps.

* Episiotomy cuts heal better than third-degree tears. However, there is disagreement as to whether they heal better than natural first- or second-degree tears.

Disadvantages:

* Episiotomy can turn an otherwise straightforward labour into a surgical event.

* Stitches can be painful for about 10 days or more after the birth, whereas with a tear there is usually less pain, often over a shorter period of time.

* Infection is a real possibility because the swollen, bruised muscles encourage bacteria to breed. This necessitates a course of antibiotics which can enter your baby's system via your breastmilk, impairing the ability of the baby's immature immune system to ward off infection.

* Some women experience the stitching-up after an episiotomy as more painful than giving birth.

* Very occasionally the wound opens up. Although it can heal by itself, many practitioners recommend re-stitching, which can be quite an ordeal.

Forceps and Vacuum Extraction

Forceps or vacuum extraction (ventouse) can be used to correct an unusual fetal position by rotating the baby's head round the right way or to provide the extra force needed to deliver the baby. However, if the baby is in a very difficult position a caesarean section may be safer for both mother and baby than a prolonged and traumatic instrumental delivery. Forceps, in particular, can cause a great deal of damage to the mother's perineum and internal organs as well as causing pain and distress to the baby. While this form of assisted delivery has its place in modern obstetrics, some observers see forceps and vacuum extraction (and caesarean section), particularly if they are unnecessary, not so much as forms of childbirth but as methods of fetal extraction.

When the mother is working with her contractions and is in an upright position, delivery rarely needs this kind of assistance. However, if the baby is genuinely in distress during the second stage of labour, forceps or vacuum extraction can be life-saving. For mothers who have severe high blood pressure, lung or heart disease, it may not be wise to become involved in vigorous bearing down. In these cases an assisted delivery is advisable.

If you have an assisted delivery as your baby is crowning (a 'lift out' delivery), you will most certainly have an episiotomy which will require an injection of a local anaesthetic to numb the whole of the birth outlet. In some cases, such as when the baby is quite high up in the birth canal (known as a 'mid-cavity' delivery), the mother will require epidural or caudal anaesthetic if she has not already had one.

For an assisted delivery you will need to be on your back with your legs supported by stirrups. You can request that your partner be allowed to stay with you, if this is what you both want. Some partners do find witnessing these kinds of deliveries upsetting, so it may be better if he or she sits near you at the top of the delivery table. With a forceps delivery, the spoon-shaped metal blades are inserted into the vagina until they grip the sides of the baby's head. Your practitioner will apply sufficient force at the handles to keep the blades from slipping as he or she pulls the baby out over the course of two or three contractions. In between contractions, your practitioner should reduce the pressure on the baby's head a little to minimize the pain and potential damage to it.

With vacuum extraction, a small suction cup made of either metal or rubber is inserted into the vagina and fitted onto the baby's scalp. It will take a few minutes for sufficient suction to build up, then your practitioner will use traction (pulling on the cord attached to the suction cup) to pull the baby out. Although a soft, rubber cup does less damage to the baby than a metal cup, it has a higher rate of failure – particularly for babies with larger heads or those whose heads are very high up in the womb. As a result, the soft cup is usually reserved for use in more 'straightforward' extractions. With vacuum extraction there is not always

Managing Labour

a need for an episiotomy because the suction cup does not take up the same amount of room in the vagina as forceps do.

Both methods have a significant failure rate – between 2 and 10 per cent for forceps and 10 and 19 per cent for ventouse.[37] If these methods fail, the baby will usually be delivered by caesarean and the mother will be left to deal with the much increased physical trauma and pain as well as feelings of sadness, depression and 'failure'.

Both methods are associated with short- and long-term problems for mothers and babies. For mothers these include perineal, cervical and vaginal tears, urinary and faecal incontinence, the feeling of prolapse and long-term pain, and a greater need for pain-killing drugs after birth. Mothers who have had assisted deliveries are also more likely to report health problems with their children, though it is not clear whether these problems are related to the traumatic method of birth or whether children delivered instrumentally do in fact suffer from more chronic complaints.[38] Babies who have been delivered instrumentally often have bruises on their faces, and sore, swollen areas on their heads. Scalp/facial injury is thought to be in the region of 9 to 51 per cent with a forceps delivery and 4 to 30 per cent with ventouse.[39] It is now known that babies feel the pain of these procedures, so this can be a particularly harsh way to enter the world, particularly if the procedure is unnecessary.

You do not have to accept an instrumental delivery if you feel it has been suggested without good reason. Certainly an arbitrary time limit on the duration of the second stage is never a sufficient reason for an assisted delivery. Provided you and your baby are coping well, less traumatic measures should be tried first, such as assuming a more upright or supported squatting position.

Advantages:

* If the mother has lost all urge and/or ability to push – often the result of augmentation and/or pain-killing drugs – an assisted delivery may be the only way to get the baby out.

* In cases of fetal distress, assisted delivery can be a life-saver.

* Mothers who suffer from debilitating conditions such as diabetes or heart or lung trouble may view an assisted delivery as preferable to the risks to their own and their baby's health of a long period of strenuous pushing.

* Ventouse is probably preferable to forceps. It is thought to cause less trauma and pain to both mother and baby.

* Forceps or ventouse can sometimes be used sparingly to correct a difficult fetal position so that the mother can go on to push the baby out herself.

Disadvantages:

* Forceps and ventouse deliveries are often the result of the arbitrary time limits which many practitioners put on the second stage of labour.

* Forceps can cause you enormous pain during and after labour. You will feel sore and bruised. Pelvic pain and painful stitches are common with these procedures.

* Many women feel a sense of disappointment and a nagging sense of failure when these instruments are used, particularly if they have not received an adequate explanation as to why they were necessary in the first place.

* There is evidence to show that babies feel the pain of assisted deliveries, and damage can result in the sensitive head and neck area.

* The bruising which babies delivered with forceps have is a sign of how hard they have been jerked around. Your baby may be cranky and unsettled for the first few days while this heals.

* There is no evidence to show whether or not vacuum extraction causes the same amount of pain as forceps to the baby, but the procedure does leave its mark. The baby may have an area of bruising and/or swelling where the suction cup was.

* Not all practitioners are skilled at using forceps. The result can be post-partum haemorrhage and damage to the internal organs, including bladder, womb and vagina. Side-effects of this can be urinary and faecal incontinence and a continual sensation of vaginal or uterine prolapse.

Caesarean Operation
In a caesarean delivery the baby, the placenta and membranes will be pulled out through a surgical incision low down in the mother's abdomen. This is known as a 'bikini line' cut. Afterwards the layers of the uterus, the muscles and the skin will be stitched and/or stapled separately. While there is no disagreement that there are far too many caesareans performed in the UK (and in fact all over the world) today, few practitioners are able to acknowledge their part in, or put a stop to, the epidemic. The caesarean rate in the UK is now at 15 per cent and rising.[40] Almost half of these are entirely unnecessary. Analysis of available data reveals that there is no correlation between the fall in perinatal deaths and the rise in caesarean rates.[41] This has led to a general agreement that a rate of around 7 per cent is both realistic and achievable, and that any rate above this ceases to

improve or make any difference in the overall outcome for mothers or babies.[42] In spite of this, the option of a caesarean is often presented to some mothers as a matter of life or death for them or their babies. What's more, there is a very strong feeling among consultants that the decision whether or not to perform a caesarean is a medical one which has nothing to do with the mother.

Both directly and indirectly, though, it has a great deal to do with all of us. The cost of unnecessary caesareans in this country can be measured both in terms of the emotional and physical damage they leave in their wake as well as in pounds and pence. Women who have caesareans suffer from more backache, constipation, depression, tiredness, insomnia, haemorrhoids and flatulence than other mothers.[43] It is also estimated that the total cost of unnecessary caesareans in this country is now in the region of £30 million a year.[44]

The most common reasons for performing a caesarean are 'failure to progress' and 'fetal distress'. It cannot be stressed strongly enough that these are highly subjective diagnoses which can be based on personal prejudices, the enforcement of artificial time limits, the administration of labour-inducing or pain-relieving drugs, and sometimes an understaffed labour ward.

In one random sample of 400 obstetricians, 47 per cent cited fear of litigation over a difficult vaginal birth as their primary reason for performing a caesarean.[45] Those who feel that the NHS offers a superior service, free from the medico-legal pressures felt by doctors in the US, should, it appears, think again. In the same survey 19 per cent said they would perform a caesarean 'because of fetal monitoring', which confirms data from other reports that EFM leads to increased caesarean rates.

Other questionable reasons for performing a caesarean include cephalopelvic disproportion, where the baby's head is considered too large or the mother's pelvis too small. This is often cited as a reason for 'failure to progress', though true cephalopelvic disproportion is not very common. If the baby is lying in a breech position many doctors consider this reason enough for an automatic caesarean. It is not. First of all, half of all breeches presenting at 32 weeks will turn before or during labour. Secondly, there is almost no reason why a normal breech baby can't be delivered vaginally. The practice of performing a caesarean under these circumstances has meant that many doctors and midwives have become completely deskilled in delivering breech babies. It is this lack of skill, rather than the inherent dangers of a breech presentation, which leads many doctors to wield the knife too soon.

True life-or-death situations with regard to mothers and babies are rare. In reality, the only circumstances in which a caesarean is necessary are fulminating pre-eclampsia, placenta praevia or placental abruption, or if the mother has a serious heart condition or kidney disease. If a mother is having an active attack of genital herpes a caesarean might also be preferred, and some practitioners believe that caesarean is the best option for a baby whose mother is HIV positive, though this is the subject of debate. When a caesarean is genuinely necessary a mother can be reassured that it is now so much a part of the routine of birth that the skill of her practitioner can be almost guaranteed.

Caesareans are not, however, a matter of routine for mothers. A caesarean is a major operation (the fact that we refer to them benignly as 'sections' rather than using the more menacing 'operations' is one of those peculiar twists of obstetric language). Mothers who have their babies delivered this way have an increased number of emotional and physical consequences to deal with. Mothers who have caesareans are four times more likely to die – from infection, haemorrhage, and inhaling their own vomit under a general anaesthetic – than mothers who do not – 40 per 100,000 as opposed to 10 per 100,000 (one American study has put the first figure at 60 per 100,000[46]). In particular, mothers who have unplanned caesareans (usually referred to as emergency caesareans, though again the definition of 'emergency' varies) are the ones who suffer the most emotional damage.[47] They often have to cope with their own feelings of bitterness, frustration, confusion, sadness, pain and sense of failure. All of which are the opposite of what they may have expected to feel about the birth of their babies.

Few carers are aware of or able to acknowledge the grief that a woman may feel at this time. Well-meaning comments that a woman should 'be happy you have a healthy baby' can produce a great deal of guilt in a woman who is plainly not happy. Guilt and grief then become a vicious circle, each feeding the other, ultimately affecting the woman's self-esteem and sometimes her ability to form a meaningful connection with her baby.

Many women never receive an adequate explanation as to why the operation was necessary in the first place. Here is where midwives can, but often fail to, help. Since it is rare for the mother or the father to be the first person to see or hold a baby delivered by caesarean, Caroline Flint sensitively advises that the day after a caesarean the midwife should go to the mother and:

> ... talk her through the caesarean section, telling her exactly how her baby was born, telling her what the baby did when he was born – whether he cried or passed urine, whether he opened his eyes, whether he whimpered, how he looked and what the people there might have said about him. It is also useful for her to have photos of the baby's birth.
>
> The woman needs to be helped to come to terms with this scar on her body, to be helped to touch it and to absorb it into herself as part of her new mother's body. Women who have had vaginal deliveries often need the same help coming to terms with their altered genitals – even if the change is so slight that an observer would not be able to see it.[48]

In addition, a caesarean has implications for any future births. Some consultants have a 'once a caesarean, always a caesarean' policy, which will more accurately be reflected in the vaginal-birth-after-caesarean (VBAC) rates of the women in their care than in the stated policy of the unit. This can make the possibility of having a normal delivery next time another long, uphill struggle. This kind of policy, once again, flies in the face of the facts. Possible rupture of the scar is usually given as the reason for repeat caesareans. Yet the incidence of rupture is minute. Some scars do rupture, but without any symptoms such as bleeding or pain. These are minor ruptures which cause no problems to mother or baby and heal by themselves. Excluding this kind of rupture, the rate of reported uterine rupture for women undergoing a trial of labour with single, normal babies is measured in fractions of a per cent, ranging from 0.09 to 0.22 per cent for women who have had the lower-segment 'bikini line' cut. To put these figures into perspective, it is estimated that the risk of a woman requiring a caesarean for true emergency conditions such as placenta praevia, cord prolapse or fetal distress is 2.7 per cent – nearly 30 times greater than the risk of uterine rupture.[49]

In spite of doctors' dire warnings, VBAC has a high success rate. A substantial review of medical literature on VBACs from 1950 to 1980 found that, of 5,325 VBACs, there was not a single maternal death related to uterine rupture. Although there were 15 fetal deaths, 12 of these were due to the rupture of a previous classical scar (an old-style cut which ran vertically up towards the navel), and only two were related to the rupture of a 'bikini' cut. Both of these occurred before 1965 in unmonitored women.[50] There is almost no physiological reason why a mother who has had a previous caesarean cannot achieve a vaginal birth the next time around. Research puts the success rate as high as 90 per cent, depending on the reasons for the mother's previous caesarean.[51] Mothers who are most likely to achieve VBACs are those whose previous caesarean was performed because the baby was in the breech position. Those who had the operation because of 'failure to progress', 'fetal distress', cephalopelvic disproportion or more than one previous caesarean may achieve a VBAC in 50 to 75 per cent of cases.[52]

The introduction of spinal anaesthesia has meant that, unlike 20 years ago when general anaesthetic was the norm, a mother who undergoes a caesarean can see her baby soon after delivery. It has also meant that partners are generally allowed to be present to provide moral support and to be the first family member to hold the baby. Today an epidural is the best form of anaesthetic in a caesarean operation, unless there is a real emergency. In spite of this, only about half of caesareans actually take place under epidural anaesthetic.[53] Because an epidural takes time to site and to take effect, in dire emergencies a general anaesthetic will be used. In extreme emergencies doctors may have to perform what is known as a 'crash section', which is a caesarean section without the aid of any anaesthetic at all. Other times doctors perform a caesarean without realizing (or unwilling to believe) that the anaesthetic has not taken effect. Women who have had caesarean operations without the benefit of anaesthetic can be traumatized for life. They may also have a difficult time convincing anyone (lawyers or doctors) that it really happened. Yet it is estimated that around 400 women a year go through this terrible ordeal.[54] If you have this experience, contact AIMS (*see Appendix C for address*), who will be able to advise you on the best way to proceed.

Some caesareans are elective, which means that the mother and/or the doctor have decided that it will be best to deliver the baby surgically on an elected date before the mother goes into spontaneous labour. One survey estimated that nearly half of the caesareans performed in one hospital with a 14 per cent caesarean rate over a six-month period were elective. Of these, 18 per cent were done at the mother's request.[55] This pattern seems to have repeated itself elsewhere, prompting doctors to claim that the rise in caesareans is justified because it is in response to women's wishes. There is very little research to enlighten us as to what may prompt a significant proportion of healthy women to ask for a caesarean and what influence, if any, their doctors may have had in the decision-making process.

Elective caesarean is rarely necessary or desirable except in circumstances where the mother's or baby's health may be severely compromised by being in labour. Elective caesareans are more often performed for the doctor's, and occasionally the mother's, convenience. Even if a caesarean is desirable or

Managing Labour

unavoidable, there is considerable evidence to show that both mother and baby can benefit from a period of spontaneous labour.[56] Certain stress hormones, known as catecholamines, are released during labour to trigger the baby's lungs to begin drying out in readiness for life in an airy environment. These hormones also stimulate the baby's liver, kidneys and digestive system to begin to function independently. Elective caesarean effectively deprives the baby of this important preparation for life in the world.

In addition, elective caesareans or those performed before the mother has reached 4-cm dilation may have implications for any subsequent births. These mothers are more likely to suffer slow or halted labours (dystocia) the next time around, increasing the possibility of having a repeat caesarean.[57] Also, an elective caesarean performed well before term is likely to cut into the thicker upper segment of the uterine muscle instead of into the thinner connective tissue near the cervix. Since the upper part of the uterus is the most active in labour, this may slightly increase the risk of uterine rupture should the mother wish to have a vaginal delivery in a subsequent birth.

To prepare for a caesarean section your pubic hair will be partially shaved off. After the anaesthesia is administered, a narrow tube called a catheter will be inserted via your urethra into the bladder to drain off urine, and an intravenous drip (dextrose and water) will be inserted into your arm to keep you hydrated. Once your abdomen has been disinfected the surgeon will make the cut. With the 'bikini line' incision the skin and uterus are cut horizontally and the abdominal muscles are torn apart vertically so that they will separate along the natural line. The rationale for this rather aggressive-sounding procedure is that it causes less trauma to the abdominal tissues and this in turn means less bleeding, less pain and better healing.

After the operation you will need some form of pain relief at least for the first 24 hours. This can be administered via pessaries in the anus, by shots of pethidine or by leaving the epidural cannula in. Generally speaking, during this time hospitals tend to leave both the urethral catheter and the glucose drip in as well. There is no evidence to show that this has any value. It will certainly make the mother feel more helpless and will restrict her movements and her efforts to establish breastfeeding. The sooner you can get up and walk to the toilet, the sooner you can negotiate to have these tubes removed. The first time you walk after a caesarean it may feel as if your abdomen is going to split open – it won't. Hold your stomach if you need to and shuffle along anyway. In fact, the earlier you can get up the better – mobility improves healing, prevents blood clots developing in the veins in the legs, and restores some sense of control.

There is no reason why you can't breastfeed your baby after a caesarean. Some hospitals take the baby away to allow the mother time to recover. You can insist that the baby be with you and that you be helped to establish breastfeeding. You may find it difficult to feed sitting up, even in a very well-supported position, but you will be able, with help, to lie on your side with the baby next to you and feed the baby this way. This is a lovely, intimate, relaxed way to feed your baby. Many caesarean mothers find that establishing successful breastfeeding is an important way of re-establishing faith in their own body's ability to function normally.

You do not have to stay in hospital after a caesarean if you don't want to. Provided you and your baby are well and you have arranged plenty of help at home, you may feel more comfortable and make a better recovery in familiar surroundings.

If your doctor suggests an elective caesarean you have the right to know exactly why, and you have the right to refuse. You also have the right to seek a second opinion. There is no reason to deny a woman a trial of labour for any but the most pressing medical reasons. If you are in labour and your practitioner suggests a caesarean, you do not have to agree. You cannot be forced, even in labour, to have an operation which you do not want. If you feel confident that your labour is progressing, however slowly, then you should be allowed to carry on.

Managing Labour

Advantages:

* Ensures the delivery of a healthy baby in cases of placenta praevia or when the baby is in a difficult position such as a transverse lie.

* Can be a life-saver for mothers with fulminating pre-eclampsia, heart condition or kidney disease.

* The operation can be performed quickly if necessary, for instance if the baby is distressed.

* The sheer number of caesareans performed each year means that your practitioner will be highly skilled in this procedure.

Disadvantages:

* A caesarean is major abdominal surgery and takes much longer to recover from than a vaginal delivery.

* Coping with the side-effects of a caesarean may make the job of coping with new motherhood more difficult.

* Babies born by caesarean have a high rate of respiratory problems at birth.

* With an elective caesarean there is a possibility that your baby will be born prematurely and therefore be less able to cope with life outside the womb.

* It is more difficult, though not impossible, to establish breastfeeding after a caesarean.

* The decision of when and if to have a caesarean is often taken out of the hands of the mother in labour.

* A mother having a caesarean may have to battle to have a vaginal birth with her next baby, if this is what she wants.

* Caesareans can affect future fertility. Caesarean mothers may find it harder to conceive next time around.

* Women who have caesareans are four times as likely to die than those who deliver vaginally.

* Rarely, the surgeon will cut too deeply and superficially damage the baby.

* Some women find the (occasionally permanent) loss of some or all feeling in the lower abdomen disturbing.

* Mothers who have caesareans find increased difficulty resuming their sex lives. Having 'failed' in the sexual act of delivering a baby, they often fear 'failure' in other sexual activities as well.

* Caesarean mothers take more medicines postnatally, including antibiotics, analgesics, anti-depressants and tranquillizers. They may also take vitamin and iron supplements. All of these substances can enter the baby's system via breastmilk and may produce ill-effects such as diarrhoea, decreased immune response, disorientation and difficulty or loss of interest in suckling.

The Third Stage of Labour

The delivery of the placenta, or afterbirth, is often relegated to an afterthought by many practitioners and mothers. In traditional cultures this third stage of labour is given more respect. After all, the placenta is the miraculous organ which has kept your baby alive and healthy for nine months. It deserves some consideration and respect.

This loss of respect for the third stage means that many practitioners see it as merely a matter of medical routine. Viewed in this way, it becomes a good excuse for another cascade of interventions which include early cutting of the cord, controlled traction of the cord to pull the placenta out and the use of syntometrine to aid the expulsion of the placenta.[58]

Delivery of the placenta can take anywhere from 5 minutes to an hour. Practitioners reason that if this stage is not actively managed, there is greater risk of retained placenta and post-partum haemorrhage. This is not, however, borne out by research. Although there is a role for the use of syntometrine in the treatment of post-partum haemorrhage, the evidence is not clear as to whether it can be considered an effective routine prophylactic (preventative) measure.[59] In spite of this many hospitals continue to administer syntometrine as a matter of course.

One of the medical profession's first interventions in this stage of labour was early cutting of the umbilical cord. This deprived the baby of vital blood, but because blood continued to be pumped out of the cut cord, did not affect the separation of the placenta. However, because it was very messy and was introduced at a time when women gave birth in their own beds, the practice of cord clamping became fashionable. Clamping the cord not only deprives the baby of blood, it sets up a counter-resistance in the placenta, delaying and sometimes preventing separation. When the blood can't flow out of the cord it collects in and behind the placenta. The longer the placenta remains undelivered, the greater the likelihood of haemorrhage because the uterus can't clamp down while the bulky placenta is inside.

Because of this, controlled cord traction was then introduced to speed things up. But pulling on the cord has many disadvantages. First, the cord can break, requiring the manual removal of the placenta under general anaesthetic or epidural. There is also a risk of pulling out an incompletely separated placenta, leaving a portion behind which will have to be removed manually, sometimes under a general anaesthetic. Finally, if the placenta has not begun to separate there is a risk of fully or partially inverting the uterus (pulling it out of the vagina).

To cope with all these possibilities, ergometrine (derived from ergot, a fungus which acts to cause muscle contractions) was introduced into third-stage management. Later, syntometrine (a powerful drug which is a combination of syntocinon and ergometrine) became popular. While the syntocinon works immediately to separate the placenta from the uterine wall, ergometrine kicks in 5 to 7 minutes later, causing further sustained contractions which act to clamp off blood vessels.

The use of these drugs has implications for both mother and baby. Many mothers report feeling nauseous. They can also experience vomiting, headaches, raised blood pressure, tinnitus, palpitations, and cramps in the back and legs.[60] Controlled cord traction and fundal pressure (pressing hard on the uterus at the placental site), used in conjunction with syntometrine, increase the risk of retained placenta and post-partum haemorrhage. This is because of the amount of stress placed on the uterus (by drugs and rough handling) and also because many practitioners, deskilled in the practice of 'expectant' third-stage management and ignorant of the physiological mechanisms of the delivery of the placenta, end up pulling on the cord before there are definite signs of separation.

For the baby there is a risk of over-transfusion. A newborn's system is designed to cope with around 120 ml of blood. The effect of syntometrine is to push the uterus into overdrive, pumping a greater volume of blood through the cord into the baby's system. This sets up a medical dilemma: when does the practitioner cut the cord? If the cord is cut early there may not be enough blood to support the baby's circulatory system. Under these circumstances its body will divert blood from elsewhere such as the respiratory system, leaving the lungs underinflated. Lowered blood volume is thought to be the cause of idiopathic respiratory distress (breathing difficulties for 'no apparent reason'). Proper lung expansion is especially crucial for preterm or low-birthweight babies, however, it is thought that even vigorous, full-term infants experience blood volume loss as a shock to the system.

If the cord is left uncut the baby can become over-transfused – sometimes doubling the amount of blood in the baby's system – putting enormous stress on its vital organs and causing jaundice. Jaundice is caused by the process of breaking down excess red blood cells. In this process a substance called bilirubin is produced which has to be excreted by the liver. If the liver is unable to cope with large amounts of bilirubin, it builds up in the blood and turns the baby's skin yellow.

The alternative to all this is a physiological third stage. This is the best way to prevent post-partum haemorrhage in mothers who have not had their labours altered by induction and/or instrumental or surgical deliveries. If the baby is put to the breast soon after birth this will release oxytocin into the mother's system which will help the placenta separate naturally. If a mother is squatting, kneeling or standing the placenta will literally fall out of her vagina aided by gravity. Provided the cord is not cut until it stops pulsating, the baby will get its full complement of blood. If the baby is not ready to feed immediately, gentle nipple stimulation can also promote the release of oxytocin.

Post-partum haemorrhage and retained placenta are not the inevitable result of labour. Every birth is not a death waiting to happen. Research into the predictive factors of third-stage problems is inconclusive and confused. There is no reason to expect problems unless there have been interventions in the delivery of your baby and the delivery of your placenta. Anaemia, known blood-clotting disorders, previous third-stage problems and multiple pregnancy may, but do not always, contraindicate a physiological third stage.

Because the delivery of the placenta is usually ignored in ante-natal education – and because the evidence is so confused – few women are aware that they have a choice. You should discuss this stage of labour well in advance with your carer. You are not obliged to accept any 'routine' policy if you don't want to. Make your preferences known verbally and in your birth plan.

It may also be of interest to note that your placenta is your property.[61] It should not be taken away without your consent, and you should be consulted about the manner of its disposal. Some hospitals still sell placentae to face cream and cosmetic manufacturers (though few will readily admit this, and the practice is now being phased out due to fear of HIV and hepatitis). Others put them, three to a bag, into the incinerator. Some women will find these options distressing and wish to dispose of their placenta themselves. Some find it helpful to create rituals such as burying it in the garden, perhaps under a new tree or shrub, to mark the birth of their baby. Others believe that eating it immediately or freezing it for future consumption is a way of getting extra iron and preventing depression.

There is no 'right' way to give birth, even at this stage. You should do whatever you feel most comfortable with. The only guideline is that you come away from the experience knowing you did what felt right for you and your baby.

6
Back to Normal?

The year after birth can be an unexpected, overwhelming rollercoaster of an experience; the physical and emotional ups and downs are surprising to every woman. There are so many positive things about being a mother, particularly during this time. There is the incomparable sensuousness of a baby – its smell, the feel of its skin next to yours, the intimacy and relaxed moments (particularly when breastfeeding is going really well). There are the little milestones – smiling, sitting up, walking, new teeth – which mark the passing months. There is the unique opportunity to rediscover the world through a child's eyes. Some women, having come through labour and birth more or less unscathed, feel more comfortable with their bodies than ever before. Some discover new emotional and spiritual strength which gives them the opportunity to redefine themselves on their own terms, instead of always in relation to somebody else's expectations. Female friendships take on a new dimension during this time too, and many women discover a new joy in forging relationships with others who are going through the same things.

Under the best circumstances in the world, the 'fourth trimester'[1] – the three months or so after birth – is a shock to the system, since no area of your life or your body remains untouched. If you have had a difficult or badly managed birth, however, the problems of the postnatal period can last much longer and be much more difficult to cope with. Either way, caught in the middle of physical and emotional upheaval many new mothers ask 'why didn't somebody tell me it would be like this?' The usual answer – 'we didn't want to put you off' – can suddenly seem more controlling than kind. Once you have a living, breathing, crying baby in your arms it becomes obvious that preserving only happy images of motherhood denies women the totality of their experience as well as the tools with which to cope during this time of enormous transition.

In our culture it is assumed that a mother will be 'back to normal' by the time of her six-week check-up. In fact, the timing of the six-week check-up does not have any intrinsic significance at all, physiologically or emotionally. It is a random time limit, the origin of which is lost in the annals of time. Ironically, this is the time when, caught up in the heady whirlwind of new parenthood and still, more or less, supported by the healthcare system, women are least likely to express dissatisfaction with themselves, their births, their care and their babies. Ask any mother how she feels about these things soon after birth and she will probably express mostly positive feelings. Ask her again at three months and she is likely to be a little more up front about all the difficulties and things which have gone, and are continuing to go, wrong.

Few practitioners follow a mother's progress for more than a few days or weeks after birth. As such, they have only a limited grasp of the concept of childbirth as a life event.[2] They will have no real idea of the impact which the things which they have said or done have had, for better or worse, on a woman's life. Even midwives, who are more mother-centred than most, tend to see pregnancy, birth and motherhood more in terms of their biological and medical aspects than as social and emotional events.[3]

Back to Normal?

Once discharged from care, a practitioner may never even think of a woman again. But surveys suggest that the opposite is true for the mother. She may literally remember her care-givers for ever. What's more, the memory of events surrounding birth, particularly a first birth, remain clear and accurate to women throughout their lives and, according to childbirth educator Penny Simkin: 'The significance [women] attach to negative events seems to intensify and increase over time, whereas the positive aspects remain consistently positive in most cases.' She concludes that women who felt supported and in control during labour are likely to feel more positive about mothering, while 'a less satisfying experience [makes] them angry and more assertive in the future, whereas others seem to [accept] a somewhat negative self-image.'[4]

Throughout this book, much of the emphasis has been on looking at birth in its wider context in order to make more appropriate choices and avoid painful consequences. The importance of this may only really begin to sink in during the postnatal period, when the problems and limitations of looking at birth as an isolated event come home to roost. Our childbirth education is going on around us all the time, even before pregnancy. Consciously or unconsciously we are all conditioned to believe that many of the routine interventions of maternity care are lifesavers and that much of the natural process is pathological. Rarely do we take the time to look critically at the consequences of these beliefs.

Women's health and well-being (or the lack of it) in the postnatal period have not benefited from much analysis. However, what has emerged is that a badly managed birth or one where intervention has been applied without good reason can lead to feelings of bitterness, depression, failure and anger as well as chronic ill-health. It can also have implications for future pregnancies. A very large study in Aberdeen of 22,948 women found that women who have caesareans are 23 per cent less likely to go on to have another baby than those who do not.[5] It remains unclear whether this is because of the secondary infertility (inability to conceive) which can be caused by a caesarean or whether fear of another caesarean influences women's decisions not to have more children.

Before birth there is a widely-held belief that women must not be told about the consequences of some of the ways in which we give birth, or about the difficulties of the post-partum period, for fear that they might react like caricatures of delicate Victorian ladies and collapse with the vapours.

After birth this belief turns into a conspiracy of silence as women become reluctant to discuss what they are going through for fear of being labelled 'ungrateful' or suspected of not 'bonding' properly with their babies. It is very unusual for a mother to initiate a consultation with a doctor, midwife or health visitor about any problems postnatally. Some keep worries to themselves, thinking that the problems are not 'bad enough' to 'bother' anyone with – even though in some cases the symptoms are painfully present every day and are detrimental to their daily activities and well-being. Some women are too embarrassed to talk about the difficulties they are experiencing because they affect the most intimate parts of their bodies and their lives. Others just passively accept their discomfort as a 'normal' part of motherhood. Inasmuch as this is true, women let themselves down very badly by allowing practitioners to continue to believe that the unacceptable is acceptable and that any pain or damage is the result of nature and not medicine.

Some symptoms, of course, are transient and are part of the natural process of birth. Others which may persist in the longer term can be the result of the many interventions which we allow to interfere with the natural process. For instance, in a study of assisted versus spontaneous vaginal birth it was shown that, while both groups complained of pain in the short term, mothers who had instrumental (forceps or ventouse) deliveries were many times more likely to need additional analgesia and physiotherapy and to suffer moderate to severe perineal discomfort afterwards. In the longer term, persistent perineal pain resulted in persistently painful intercourse. Mothers whose babies were instrumentally delivered also had more long-term worries about their babies' health. They were more likely to perceive problems and worry that these were related to the way the baby was delivered.[6]

Birth is not an illness, but, given the number and the nature of interventions which women are currently subjected to, it can lead to illness. One mother whose birth included pethidine, an epidural, a large episiotomy and a forceps delivery wrote of her postnatal experience this way:

> I have paid £200 in osteopath fees to reduce the back pain that came as soon as the pain killing effects of the epidural wore off. I have seen my GP for neuralgia in my feet. When I get up from sitting for any length of time, the pain is so bad I sometimes find myself hobbling like an old woman ... After six months of agony, I saw my GP who said the wound [episiotomy] hadn't healed properly and needed treatment. The gynaecologist I was referred to disagreed. He said I was frigid. The anaesthetist who sited my epidural dismissed claims that my backache was a problem as nonsense.[7]

The response of her carers is all too typical. It's the woman's fault. Her wound didn't heal properly, *not* her doctor or midwife made a botched job of repairing a (possibly unnecessary) episiotomy. She was frigid, *not* she was exhausted and in pain after a badly managed and difficult birth. Having reached the point where the physical damage done and the resulting emotional fall-out is beyond anything which medicine can heal, some practitioners will resort to telling women that what they are experiencing is simply a product of fantasy or neurosis. It takes a strong and supported woman to stand up to this kind of defensive finger-pointing. The mother mentioned above, ironically also a nurse, concluded that women need fundamental information on the consequences of modern childbirth and the reality of the postnatal period. I agree. Without this information women can't be said to be making informed choices or, where necessary, exercising the right of informed refusal.

Study after study confirms that stories like this are not at all unusual. Women suffer a great deal more than we ever seem to acknowledge after birth. The results of one large study of 11,701 women who gave birth in one Birmingham hospital between 1978 and 1985 made startling reading. It concluded that nearly half of all mothers developed a wide spectrum of *totally new* physical problems after childbirth.[8] Based on their sample the authors estimate that 18.9 per cent of mothers who have an epidural, and 10.5 per cent of those who do not, suffer from backache. Overall, 4 per cent endure headaches, 8 per cent experience neck and shoulder pains, 11 per cent develop stress incontinence and 4 per cent frequency incontinence, 5 per cent get haemorrhoids, 9 per cent suffer from depression and 12 per cent from extreme fatigue. Later, summing up their findings in a medical journal, the authors concluded that for postnatal care to be truly effective it should include health checks for the mother throughout the first year, in the same way that health checks are performed on the baby.[9]

Sadly, when assessing health after birth there is a tendency to separate a woman's body from her emotions, leaving one of the most common experiences of this period, depression, without cause and without meaning. It is not unusual for a new mother to be depressed. Practitioners often make the distinction between what they call the 'baby blues', which many women experience around four days after the birth, and the persistent unhappiness which goes on for much longer. We live in a world where we are all encouraged to keep a tight rein on our 'negative' emotions and where being happy is indicative of being normal and healthy. Because of this, depression is one of the least well-understood, and least well-tolerated, emotional states.

The term 'postnatal depression' is very misleading. It suggests a specific type of emotional disturbance, distinct from other types of depression. This is not the case. Depression can occur at any time, in anyone, but is most likely to occur during times of personal upheaval. Severe depression is rare (occurring in only 1 to 2 per cent of women), but may put both mothers and their

Back to Normal?

babies at risk and should be monitored within the community by health visitors and doctors. However, to presume that all mothers should be happy with their lot is unrealistic. It may even be that depression has a real and valid role to play in the early days of motherhood.

Depression, as experienced by between 10 and 20 per cent of women after birth, can be part of a legitimate grieving process. Once your baby arrives you may need time to adjust if, for instance, it wasn't the boy or girl you had hoped for or did not look as you might have imagined. You will also need time to adjust to a body which may not feel, look or smell like your body at all. Your once firm abdomen may feel boggy and slack. You may be leaking – milk, blood, urine, sweat and occasionally tears. It may be difficult and uncomfortable to stay in one position for a long time. You may be surprised at the way you smell after giving birth. Post-partum blood is very sweet and pungent and this, mixed with the smell of breastmilk, can end up being one of your most powerful memories of the first weeks after childbirth.

New mothers may also grieve for their 'old selves' – the one which had a reason to get dressed before noon, could stay up late, come and go as she pleased, eat a meal uninterrupted, go window-shopping or to a Sunday matinee at the cinema. The one who felt confident in her work, experienced days which had a beginning, middle and end, and who received tangible rewards for a job well done. Unbeknownst to many women before they give birth, motherhood offers none of these things.

Often doctors and health visitors faced with a depressed woman will try to reassure her that it's only her hormones (either she has too many, too few, or the right ones in the wrong combination!). Leaflets targeted at new mothers sometimes define depression as feeling unhappy 'for no reason at all', or reassure new mothers that their feelings of loss, frustration and inadequacy 'usually have no foundation'. The implication is that depression in the postnatal period simply descends on a woman out of the blue – a sort of emotional or hormonal pirate which needs blasting out of the water, usually with a course of anti-depressants.

Childbirth itself does not increase a woman's chances of becoming depressed. Nor has research into the predictive factors for depression at this time produced any clear consensus. What has produced results, however, are the studies which look into the type of birth a woman experiences and its subsequent effect on her mood. In one Norwegian survey of women who gave birth in hospital, 64 per cent reported a feeling of loss of control during childbirth. More than two-thirds of these women exhibited signs of depression soon after birth. There was also a connection between feelings of depression and anxiety during the last week before birth, receiving little support from the hospital staff and 'unmet needs in relation to the midwives'.[10] The authors concluded that modern obstetric practice and hospital procedures, combined with the absence of psychological support, can directly affect a woman's mood post-partum.

Figures closer to home tell a similar story: 60 per cent of women who give birth in hospital experience depression, as opposed to only 16 per cent of those who give birth at home.[11] A high rate of depression is also associated with emergency caesareans.

At the moment, postnatal checks rarely include a detailed history of the birth itself, nor do they concentrate much on the emotional state of the mother – the assumption being that if both mother and baby are alive everything must have gone well. Simply *surviving* the process, however, is not enough. Childbirth should leave women at least as healthy as they were before pregnancy.[12] Many more sensitive observers are now recommending that we re-think postnatal check-ups to make them more emotionally, as well as physically, orientated. In the mean time, women must not confuse acknowledging their difficulties with somehow not loving their babies. A mother who is experiencing physical or emotional problems will still, generally, love her baby. But she may not *enjoy* her baby or her life, or indeed love herself, as much as she might otherwise.

There are other unexpected changes after birth which are widely experienced, but rarely discussed. Sex after childbirth –

or the lack of it – is one of the most studiously ignored issues of the post-partum period. Ante-natal classes may hint that you will feel 'a bit tired' for 'a few weeks' afterwards, but otherwise avoid the issue altogether. If sex is mentioned it is usually in the context of pelvic floor exercises (when you get to this point, you will be heartily sick of hearing about pelvic floor exercises and how they are a panacea for every mother's ills). After birth, doctors, midwives and health visitors, faced with a woman who has lost interest in sex, dogmatically recommend that if she tries out different sexual positions, encourages her partner to pleasure her without penetration (and keeps doing her pelvic floor exercises), all will be well. This advice – whether the product of embarrassment or ignorance – ignores an important basic fact: most women simply don't feel like having sex for a very long time after giving birth.

Research bears this out: one survey showed that only 50 per cent of mothers were still interested in sex after birth. Of those women who were still sexually active after birth, '...a staggering 60 per cent either make love for their partner's sake or because they can't tell him they don't want to.'[13] Another survey, by the NCT, revealed similar results: around 52 per cent of women lost interest in sex after having a baby.[14]

The reasons why are complex and varied. Once again, the way a woman gives birth can have an impact. Pain and exhaustion after a long and difficult labour, forceps delivery, episiotomy or caesarean operation can decrease a woman's desire for sex. When combined with the endless routine and unrelenting intimacy which a baby demands of its mother, the relative isolation in which most mothers function, dissatisfaction with the way her body looks, lack of help with household chores, feelings of loss of identity and/or depression, it's easy to see how sex can drop to the bottom of a woman's list of priorities.

After tiredness, a sore perineum is the most common complaint of new mothers.[15] As many as 15 per cent of women will still have a painful perineum up to three years after birth, regardless of whether or not they had an episiotomy.[16] However, if you have had an assisted delivery, have torn or had an episiotomy (particularly under an epidural, where there is a tendency for practitioners to make stitches too tight), intercourse is much more likely to be chronically painful, sometimes for years afterwards. In the short term, women who have had assisted deliveries (with ventouse or forceps) are twice as likely to experience perineal pain (84 per cent as opposed to 42 per cent).[17]

Interestingly, although some 25 per cent of women in our civilized Western culture will tear during labour, in less developed countries tearing of the perineum is almost unheard of.[18] This is because mothers in these cultures do not give birth against the clock, nor are they encouraged to enter into vigorous pushing during labour. This allows the perineum time to stretch naturally to accommodate the baby's head. In the light of this it would seem that the best way to avoid chronic perineal pain, and its consequences for our intimate relationships, is to avoid situations which lead to an episiotomy or a tear in the first place.

Unfortunately, a woman who goes along to her doctor to complain of painful intercourse may not get much help. In fact, sometimes her husband gets more of the doctor's sympathy – 'Poor fellow, we need to get you sorted out for his sake.' Advice columns in magazines have taken this attitude on board and often counsel a woman to take action – the implication being that the 'problem' is hers and that she should be striving, diligently, every day to overcome it. Their 'experts' write: 'go out to dinner together', 'put yourself in the mood with a hot bath in aromatherapy oils', or 'pamper your husband with a nice back rub.' While researching this book I came across an American publication which, crudely and rather callously, recommends that for women who are experiencing painful intercourse the answer is simple: 'Medicate, Lubricate and Inebriate.'[19] Couples who take this kind of advice to heart, believing that any day now things will get back to normal, can end up feeling terribly betrayed.

Although more and more practitioners are becoming aware of the realities of the post-partum period, few feel equipped to help women deal with them. Because medical education makes them action-orientated, they end up prescribing remedial measures which either don't help or, in the case of drugs or surgical procedures, cause even more debilitating side-effects. Few would consider a sincere apology or shouldering some of the blame for the way things have turned out as a starting point, though this kind of acknowledgement can often facilitate the healing process.

Fewer still would feel comfortable with the idea of using active listening and support while the normal ups and downs of the postnatal period take their course, or of giving women 'permission' to follow their instincts or to lose interest in sex for as long as it takes after birth. But this seems to be precisely what is needed. Sometimes helpful advice and sure-fire solutions are just another form of intervention, a way of constructing a reality which the professional feels comfortable with but which ultimately has nothing to do with the reality of a woman's life.

Practitioners must also avoid the temptation to collaborate with women's profound need to justify the interventions used on them during birth. This can be a difficult idea to take on board, since the belief in the rightness of many interventions is inextricably tied up with many practitioners' sense of professional self-esteem. A woman's ability to justify the most unwarranted interventions must be viewed in part as a self-protective measure. To believe that intervention was necessary, either to improve on a dysfunctional Nature or to counter an act of God, is to make the side-effects bearable. To accept that they were not is, at least in the short term, to lose faith, confidence, hope and a sense of sovereignty at a time when these things may already be at an all-time low. However, it can do more damage in the longer term (to a woman's self-esteem and her perception of birth and her baby) to encourage her to believe in her head what she may know in her heart to be untrue.

Ante-natal classes could usefully (but rarely do) address some of these issues. Instead they seem to prefer to accentuate the positive. But the joys of new motherhood are self-evident – nobody needs to be told what's good about being a mother. Few women who are enjoying themselves and their babies will consult a book or a magazine to find out if what they are experiencing is 'normal'. However, women in pain – physical or emotional – need acknowledgement, practical help, reassurance and freedom from the guilt which arises from the belief that their problems are somehow their 'fault'.

Instead of teaching women how to breathe (as if they weren't breathing before they became pregnant), rehearsing drills for coping with contractions, or showcasing the technological wonders of the hospital environment, ante-natal groups could orientate themselves more towards empowering women, informing them of their rights and choices and being honest about what lies ahead. There is an urgent need for ante-natal education to move away from being task-orientated and more towards being process-orientated.

Finally we all need to let go of the idea of getting 'back to normal'. Pregnancy, birth and motherhood move us further along on life's continuum. They challenge us to create a new normality. After you have given birth you can't go back, you can only go forward. Unfortunately, the dearth of information about what lies ahead and the resulting fear of the unknown makes many women feel as if it might be safer to try and 'get back' to familiar territory. But once you have a baby, *your body will never be the same, your emotions will never be the same, the priorities in your life and the way you apportion your time and energy will never be the same.*

It takes awareness, skill, maturity and a great deal of patience to negotiate this time well. Like any major change of life, the period of adjustment varies between individuals and the success of the adjustment depends on the amount of support you have around you, and especially your own willingness to make the change in the first place.

Appendix A
Complaining About Care

Women, in particular, seem to find it very difficult to complain. Meetings with authority often result in a disintegration of a woman's confidence in her own authority. Nevertheless, the best time to complain about minor transgressions – such as rudeness, painful examinations, disregard for your birth plan or your wishes, an unhelpful or condescending attitude from your carer – is immediately. Don't wait until later when you are all wound up and/or your practitioner can't recall the incident. If the person you are dealing with takes no notice, you can ask to see the senior person on duty. Being assertive and making your point in the moment (or as soon as possible) is a way of defining boundaries and may keep little issues from turning into very big ones later. It sends a strong signal to those around you that you will not tolerate certain types of behaviour and/or that you have strong views about your care. Often it only takes one well-placed comment to ensure that staff behave themselves and act in a more professional and courteous manner toward you.

Serious Complaints

Sometimes there are more serious issues at stake. If your care continues to be sub-standard or causes you distress, or if you or your baby have been damaged in any way, you *must* complain through official channels. You have a right to complain and, some would argue, you have a duty to complain. If a practitioner is abusive or negligent and you don't complain you are leaving him free to treat the next woman (and baby) who comes along in the same unsatisfactory way.

You should be aware that the complaint procedures in Britain are unnecessarily complex and occasionally intimidating. There are, however, moves afoot to streamline the procedure. These are due to come into effect in April 1996 and at the time of writing have not been finalized. You are, therefore, advised to seek guidance either from your local Community Health Council (CHC) or, if they are not very helpful, Association for Improvements in the Maternity Services (AIMS; *see page 262 for address*) – a national organization which helps many women each year with their complaints about maternity care.

Before you complain, *and before you tell anybody that you are going to complain,* get hold of all your medical records. You do not have to give a reason why you want them. These should include copies of your GP's notes, your hospital case notes, any computerized records the hospital holds and, if appropriate, your child's case notes and computerized records. Get all of these, because the notations about your care made in them don't always agree. You have the right to access to these under the Access to Health Records Act 1991 and the Data Protection Act 1987 (*see page 117*).

Occasionally, women who have not got hold of their notes beforehand have found that some or all of their records have mysteriously disappeared, or been altered, making it many times more difficult to argue their cases. If you are carrying your own notes, make copies. If you are not carrying your own notes make sure you get copies on your discharge from hospital or, if you have had your baby at home, from your midwife before she discharges you from her care 10 days after the birth.

Once you are in possession of your notes you must check them to see if they tally with your memory of the situation. You may be dispirited to see how little is actually written in them. Events which loom large in your memory are sometimes hardly given any consideration by your practitioner.

Having done this you might want to write down or tape-record your memory of events. Make a note of dates, times, the people who were present, in fact every detail you can remember. Get your partner, or whoever was with you at the time, to do the same. You can then check to see if your recollections match up. Having done this you are in a much better position to consider making your complaint.

Although it is best to make your complaint as soon as possible after the fact, some women simply don't feel in a fit state to do this immediately after birth. However, there is a suggestion that new rules will provide, at most, a six-month window from the time of the incident for you to lodge your complaint. If this is the case it is important to get an initial letter in, even if you do not detail your complaint there and then. You could, for instance, write to say that you were very dissatisfied with your care and, while you are too ill to detail the events now, you wish it to go on record that you are complaining and will detail your complaint at a later date.

Often women suppress bad experiences or try to convince themselves that it wasn't that bad, in order to get on with the demanding business of caring for themselves, their babies and their families. Memories of bad care do not, however, go away that easily. Often they come back at night or when you are alone, and can be totally overwhelming. Don't underestimate the therapeutic effect of complaining. Getting your complaint off as soon as you feel able to can begin or aid the much-needed healing process.

Many professionals fail to see complaints as valuable and necessary to their continued professional development. Instead they see them as attacking and a bit of a nuisance. Doctors and midwives are often genuinely perplexed by women's complaints because they have been so strongly conditioned to believe that they only ever act in the best interests of their patients. Women who complain are often treated like neurotic whingers who just need to be humoured until they give up or become too worn down by the effort.

GPs

Make your complaint to the General Manager of the Family Health Services Authority (FHSA). The address will be in the phone book and also on your medical card. Since the FHSA will not investigate any complaints which are not about breaches of contract, you should always include a paragraph which says something like 'I would like you to investigate my complaint about Dr ____, who I believe is in breach of his/her terms of service.' If you are not up to complaining yourself, you can get someone to write on your behalf.

If the FHSA decides to pursue your complaint, a date will be made for your case to be heard by a committee of medical and lay people. You can put your case yourself or have someone (a friend, your partner) there to help you. Sometime afterwards you will receive a copy of the committee's findings and, if your case is proved, the GP may be disciplined. You cannot receive compensation from the committee but you can claim back expenses. If you disagree with the decision, you have the right to appeal to the Secretary of State for Health. If you are unhappy with the way the FHSA handled your case (in other words, with the administrative process), write to the Health Service Commissioner (known as the Ombudsman; *see page 270 for address*) and ask for an investigation.

Hospitals

If you are unhappy with the care which you have received from a doctor or midwife in hospital, you should write to the District General Manager (if the hospital is an NHS Trust, complain to

Complaining About Care

the Chief Executive). You can get the address from the hospital where you've had your baby or from your local CHC. At the time of writing there is a one-year time limit for lodging complaints of this nature, but check to make sure this has not changed. If you put in a complaint outside that time it will still be investigated, but the official complaints procedure will not necessarily be followed.

You will need to send copies of your complaint to other relevant parties such as the Chair of the Regional Health Authority, the Chair of the District Health Authority and, if complaining about a midwife, to the Supervisor of Midwives at the hospital. If you get nowhere complaining at the local level, the next step is to take your complaint to the various national professional bodies.

Complaints about professional misconduct of medical staff (GPs, obstetricians, junior staff) should be made to the General Medical Council (GMC). You should send copies to the Chair of the Regional Health Authority, your CHC, and to the practitioner concerned. The GMC does not have a good record of upholding complaints against doctors. However, by lodging your complaint at both local and national levels, you have put it 'on the record'. Should another complaint arise against the same practitioner your case will add to the weight of evidence against him or her.

Complaints about midwives, health visitors and nurses should be made to the United Kingdom Central Council for Nursing, Midwifery and Health Visiting (UKCC; *see page 271 for address*). If a preliminary investigation finds that there is a case to answer, your case will be referred to the Professional Conduct Committee. If the matter is sufficiently serious they have the power to suspend or strike the practitioner off or take other disciplinary action. Make sure you send copies of all your letters to the Supervisor of Midwifery or Director of Nursing Services (whichever is appropriate). They will need to know that you are taking your complaint further and kept informed of its progress. Often Health Authorities will only investigate your complaint on the condition that you do not intend to take legal action. This is actually a form of intimidation. No one can force you to refrain from taking legal action if, having pursued your complaint through the system, you do not feel you have received a satisfactory answer.

With any complaint you are making it is important to send out lots of copies. Complaints have a strange way of getting lost in the system. The more people who know you are complaining, the more likely it is that your complaint will be taken seriously and dealt with swiftly. Therefore, it is wise, in addition to those bodies listed above, to send copies to your MP, the Chair of your local CHC and also to the Chair of AIMS. Always keep copies of everything you write for your own reference.

If your complaint is not upheld at the local level you can still appeal. You should write to the group who heard your case that you are not satisfied with the decision and that you wish to take the matter further. Enquire to whom you should direct your appeal and ask for details of the options open to you now. These differ between professional bodies.

If any of the national professional bodies do not uphold your complaint, you can ask for a judicial review (in other words, pursue the matter through the courts). You must do this within three months of the final decision. Under certain circumstances you can get legal aid for this. Be aware that a judicial review is a major step, not to be undertaken lightly, which can cost a great deal of money.

Taking Legal Action

Very few people have the energy or motivation to pursue their doctors through the courts. However, for those who have been through the official system and have failed to get any satisfaction it may seem the only option. In her book *Who's Having Your Baby?*, Beverley Lawrence Beech points out that the medical profession considers every complainant a potential litigant, and so does everything possible to dissuade him or her from continuing with the complaint. In so doing, they force complainants into a position where litigation is the only way to get satisfaction.[1] Research from the US, where medical litigation is a way of life, suggests that those doctors who get sued the most are those who rush their consultations, who do not offer advice or explain the reasons for tests, who ignore their clients and who cannot be reached by phone.[2]

You should not consider legal action until you have considered whether all of the possibilities within the official complaints procedure would serve you better. Once you take up legal action, access to the Ombudsman is denied you; the Health Authority will not investigate your complaint if there are legal proceedings.

If you are not sure whether you have a case you should contact AIMS. Advisors there will be able to tell you whether, judging from their experience, you have a good case. You should also contact the Association for Victims of Medical Accidents (AVMA; *see page 270 for address*), an organization which advises patients who want to take legal action. AVMA is a voluntary organization who will be able to tell you, first, whether you have a case, and if so, where you can find a sympathetic and skilled solicitor in your area. If you are thinking of taking legal action it is vital that you find a lawyer who is skilled and knowledgeable in medical law. Loyalty to the pleasant man who did your will or your conveyancing may cost you your case.

Your lawyer will need to see your copies of all the relevant paperwork first – case notes, co-operation cards, X-rays etc., and should not make a pronouncement about your case until he or she has reviewed these things.

As noted earlier in this section, the Health Authority will often say that they will not investigate a complaint if you are taking legal action. However, there is no reason why the Health Authority cannot investigate those aspects of your care which are not the subject of litigation. If your Health Authority becomes too entrenched in this attitude and refuses to investigate these matters, you can, and should, complain to the Ombudsman.

Legal action against doctors does not have a good record in the UK. It is interesting to note that judges are as reluctant to question the clinical judgement of doctors as the rest of us (even though they are not shy about sticking their oar into other complex areas such as multinational corporate fraud or the embezzlement of some rock star's multi-millions). In over 70 per cent of cases the judge will find for the defence (the medical profession).[3]

When faced with a woman who is complaining about her maternity care, professionals often respond with an attitude which says, 'You have a healthy baby. Why are you complaining?' As has been noted elsewhere in this book, the fact that you and your baby are alive does not necessarily mean that all is well. If you are unhappy you have the right to complain. In cases where you and/or your baby are manifestly unwell or if your baby has died as a result of negligent care, you have every reason to make a complaint or take legal action.

Some doctors bank on the fact that mothers are too exhausted and overwhelmed after birth (or just grateful to have survived) even to think about complaining. Or they are arrogant enough to believe that no mere mother would challenge their professional expertise, or that even if she does, the panel of other doctors who judge these complaints will be loathe to condemn a peer. Many rely on the fact that in our society doctors are on the receiving end of often unshakeable good faith and a disproportionate amount of trust.

It is very difficult for a pregnant woman to complain. When you are pregnant the last thing you may have the strength for is doing battle out in the world. And it can be difficult not to get tied up in knots by the 'logic' of others.

It is very difficult to complain when you have a small baby. Your energy levels are low and time is not your own. Letters have to be written, copies made, replies received and more letters written and copied. Complaining about health care can be a full-time job. Yet, we must complain, even if official procedures are designed to discourage all but the most determined and energetic. It is only by complaining, naming names and challenging outmoded and, in some cases, downright dangerous practices that things will begin to change.

Appendix B
Maternity Rights and Benefits

Your Rights at Work

It sometimes comes as a shock to women that they do have a number of rights at work when they are pregnant and after they have given birth. Unfortunately, the rights and benefits system is unnecessarily complicated and there are a lot of grey areas. Trying to make sense of it can make you feel as if you are going crazy. Bear in mind that it's the system which is crazy, not you. Don't let information which can at first seem difficult to grasp discourage you from finding out more about your statutory rights at work.

Knowing your rights and asserting them at work are often two different things. Since a large proportion of women are in part-time or low-paid work and their families depend on their earnings, many feel it is best not to rock the boat. However, things like time off for ante-natal appointments, maternity leave and job protection are not a luxury, but a necessity. They are also the law. Britain currently has the worst record in the EU for the way it treats mothers who are employed. If women do not let employers know that they want these things and insist that they be provided, the issue of improving conditions for pregnant women and mothers will simply never be addressed.

Depending on your contract of employment you may have contractual rights as well as statutory ones. If your contract of employment gives you a contractual right to maternity leave or absence as well as the statutory right, you may take advantage of whichever is, in any particular respect, more favourable to you. For example, if your contract allows you more time off or less advance notification of your intent to take leave, you may follow the contractual scheme in these respects.

The information here is intended merely as an overview. You are strongly encouraged to seek advice from your union (if you belong to one) or a local law centre or Citizen's Advice Bureau if you need clarification about where you stand.

Time Off for Ante-natal Appointments
Ante-natal care is defined as medical examinations as well as parentcraft and relaxation classes. Regardless of how long you have been employed in a particular job, no employer can reasonably refuse you time off for these appointments.

All time off for these appointments must be paid at your normal rate of pay.

Except for your first appointment, you may need to produce a medical certificate confirming your pregnancy and some proof of your appointments such as an appointment card or other document.

If your employer denies you your normal rate of pay or refuses you time off, or if you feel you have been dismissed or made redundant because you have sought time off, you can take your case to an Industrial Tribunal.

Changing Your Job
If while you are pregnant your job becomes unsuitable for you, for instance because it involves exposure to harmful substances or heavy lifting or night work, you are entitled to:

Maternity Rights and Benefits

have your working conditions temporarily changed to remove you from the perceived risk, *or*

be offered another job at the same rate of pay and the same level of skill, *or*

if another job cannot be found for you, you should be offered maternity suspension (paid leave) for as long as is necessary to protect your health and that of your baby. See 'Getting Back To Work' (*page 254*) for more details on maternity suspension.

Losing Your Job

It is unlawful for your employer to dismiss you, or select you for redundancy in preference to other comparable employees, because you are pregnant or because you have given birth during your statutory maternity leave period. This special protection can under certain circumstances apply for up to four weeks after your statutory maternity leave. These rights apply regardless of your length of service.

Unfortunately many employers disregard the law and in reality it is estimated that around 4,000 or more women do lose their jobs every year because they are pregnant or have given birth. It can be very difficult to prove that you have been dismissed on these grounds. However, if you feel you might have a case you should seek advice from your union (if you are a member of one) as you may be able to take your case to an Industrial Tribunal. You have the right to a written explanation as to why you have been dismissed regardless of whether or not you request one and regardless of your length of service.

Maternity Leave

All pregnant employees are entitled to a period of at least 14 weeks maternity leave. This applies regardless of length of service or hours of work. The maternity leave period lasts:

until 14 weeks after the date on which it started, *or*

until two weeks after the date of childbirth, if this is later than 14 weeks after the date on which it started, *or*

if the employee works in a factory, until four weeks after the date of childbirth, if this is later than 14 weeks after the date on which it started, *or*

until some later date, if there exists another statutory requirement which prohibits the employee from working due to the fact that she has recently given birth.

In order to take advantage of maternity leave you must notify your employer of the following things at least *21 days* before you intend to start taking maternity leave and/or receiving statutory maternity pay (SMP):

the fact that you are pregnant, the expected week of your child's birth and (if you want to and you qualify for it) the fact that you intend to exercise the right to return to work after the additional maternity absence period (see below).

the date on which you wish to start taking your maternity leave (and/or receiving your SMP). You may give this notice after you have notified your employer of your pregnancy if you wish. This date must be no earlier than the beginning of the eleventh week before the expected week of childbirth.

It is best to confirm these things in writing to your employer, whether or not the employer requests you to do so. You will usually be asked to confirm the expected date of childbirth with a form Mat B1 (which can be obtained from your doctor or midwife). Your employer cannot start paying your SMP until this form has been received.

Maternity Rights and Benefits

During your maternity leave you have a statutory right to continue to benefit from all the terms and conditions of your employment, except a wage. Whether or not you continue to receive a wage remains a matter for negotiation and agreement on a voluntary or contractual basis.

This means that you will continue to accrue holiday entitlement and your employer must continue to pay any pension contributions on your behalf. You are also entitled to continue to participate in company share schemes, be reimbursed for professional subscriptions, use the company car and mobile phone (unless these are designated for business use only) and other perks such as health club membership. Whether or not you continue to pay pension contributions depends on the individual scheme and whether or not you are receiving any SMP or any contractual remuneration. If you are, you will be treated as having a wage and will be asked to continue to pay only on the amount of money you are actually receiving.

As you are still employed during maternity leave this period counts towards your period of continuous employment for the purposes of assessing seniority, pension rights and other personal length-of-service payments such as pay increments. If you are denied any of these rights you can pursue the matter through the civil courts, just as if you were still at work. You could also resign and make a complaint of unfair dismissal to an Industrial Tribunal. This can be a long, drawn-out process, though; you are strongly advised to take professional advice from a local law centre or Citizen's Advice Bureau before taking any action of this kind.

If you give birth before your expected date, your maternity leave period automatically starts on the date of birth. As soon as is reasonably practicable you must notify your employer of the date of birth.

If you are absent from work due to an illness which is not pregnancy-related you are entitled to take sick leave and may receive Statutory Sick Pay/Sickness Benefit until your maternity leave period begins. If you are absent from work due to a pregnancy-related reason, your maternity leave period will begin automatically on the first day of absence following the beginning of the sixth week before the expected week of childbirth. As soon as is reasonably practicable you must notify your employer of the reason for your absence.

If you are dismissed or you resign before the notified start date of your maternity leave you will lose the right to maternity leave, but your employer will still have to pay all of your SMP if you are entitled to it. Payment will begin in accordance with your notified date or, if the dismissal or resignation has taken place before you have notified a date, the 11th week before the expected week of childbirth or the first week after employment ends (whichever is the later).

You do not have to give your employer advance notice if you intend to return to work immediately after the end of your maternity leave. But if you intend to return before the end of your maternity leave period you must give your employer *7 days'* notice.

Maternity Absence
Some women qualify for an *additional* period of maternity absence. If you have worked for the same employer for a continuous period of two years up to the 11th week before your expected week of childbirth, you qualify for this extra leave, which lasts from the end of your maternity leave period until the end of the 28th week after the week in which you give birth.

There is a loophole in the law which says that if you work for a firm which employs five or fewer employees you may not necessarily be entitled to maternity absence. There are, however, exceptions. For instance, if you work in a shop which has five employees but that shop is part of a larger chain employing hundreds, your entitlement will be assessed in relation to the overall number of employees and not just those at your branch.

Your employer is entitled to write to you at any time from 21 days before the end of your maternity leave and ask for written confirmation of your intention to return. Your employer's letter

Maternity Rights and Benefits

must include notification that if you fail to reply *within 14 days* you will lose your right to return.

You are obliged to write to your employer at least *21 days* before your return to confirm the date of your exact date of return.

Unlike during your maternity leave period, there is no statutory requirement for your employment to continue during maternity absence. Nor is there any statutory requirement for you to continue to benefit from any of your normal terms and conditions of employment during this time. It will be up to you to negotiate these with your employer. Your job is not protected during this time, so again it will be up to you to negotiate with your employer about this.

This period of maternity absence can be extended by an additional period of up to four weeks due to a medically-certified illness. You must give your employer advance notification of your intention to take this option and send a copy of a medical certificate stating that you will be incapable of returning to work on the previously agreed date.

Maternity Benefits

Astonishingly few women actually qualify for maternity benefits. The system seems designed to refuse all but the high-paid, long-serving employee. Since 30 per cent of women are in part-time employment (representing some 80 per cent of all part-time workers) this can only be very discouraging news. All women qualify for maternity leave, but the catch is that not all qualify for the statutory maternity payment which would make exercising the right to take leave practicable. Without this money to support them, many women endanger their health and that of their baby by working right up to the last minute and returning to work soon after their babies are born.

It would be wonderful to have a government which put its money where its mouth was, investing in family from the very beginning by providing statutory maternity leave child care on a par with the rest of Europe. For instance, in Italy mothers get two

Every Woman's BirthRights

months off before birth and three months off after on 80 per cent pay, with the option of six months extra parental leave on 30 per cent pay. In France women have six weeks off before birth and 10 weeks after on 84 per cent pay, with the option of unpaid parental leave until the child is three, at which point he or she can enter one of the country's full-time nurseries.

Sweden, however, provides the gold standard to which we should look for inspiration. There, men and women are given 50 days parental leave. Mothers are given 18 months maternity leave per child on 90 per cent pay. Each year parents get 90 days' paid leave to care for sick children until the child is 12 years old, and also two days per year for visits to nursery or school. Parents also have the option of working six-hour days until the child is 8 years old. Britain, by contrast, has the most part-time workers but the lowest provision for maternity pay in the EU. At the moment the impetus for change is coming solely from charitable organizations, such as the Maternity Alliance and Working for Childcare, enlightened employers, and mothers.

If you are on a very low income, you may, aside from the benefits listed below, qualify for Income Support, Family Credit or One-parent Benefit. Your local Social Security office or Citizens Advice Bureau can advise you.

Statutory Maternity Pay (SMP)

If you are pregnant or have just given birth you are entitled to a maximum of 18 weeks' SMP if:

> you have worked for your employer for a continuous period of at least 26 weeks ending with the 15th week before the expected week of childbirth, *and*

> you have average weekly earnings in the eight weeks up to and including the qualifying week (15th week), or equivalent period if you are paid monthly, equal to £58 – in other words, the lower earnings limit for National Insurance contributions.

Maternity Rights and Benefits

You must give your employer at least *21 days* notice that you wish to receive SMP. You can work right up until the date your baby is born and still retain your right to the full 18 weeks' SMP.

Statutory Maternity Pay is paid by your employer regardless of whether you intend to return to work or not, and regardless of whether you leave work before you want your SMP to start.

SMP is a weekly benefit which is usually paid in the same way and at the same time as your normal wages. The first six weeks of SMP are paid at 90 per cent of your average weekly earnings (or at the SMP flat rate of £54.55 per week, if this is higher). The remaining weeks are paid at the SMP flat rate.

Maternity Allowance
Women who are not entitled to SMP but have worked and paid National Insurance contributions in 26 out of the 66 weeks prior to the week before the expected week of birth are entitled to claim a maximum of 18 weeks' MA from the Benefits Agency. You can receive Maternity Allowance if:

you are employed but do not qualify for SMP, or if you have recently been employed, or if you are self-employed.

Claims should be made using the form MA1 available from the ante-natal clinic and the Benefits Agency. A qualifying employee can work right up to the date her baby is born and still retain her right to the full 18 weeks of Maternity Allowance. There are two rates of MA: £54.55 per week for those who were employed in the qualifying week (the 15th week before birth) and £47.35 for those who were not employed or were self-employed in the qualifying week.

Child Benefit
If you have been living in Britain for at least six months, you can claim Child Benefit. This is a weekly benefit paid from the week of birth for each child under 18 and does not depend on National Insurance contributions. For the first child the rate is £10.80 per

week and for each subsequent child the rate is £8.85. This is payable in weekly or four-weekly instalments, either by order book or directly into your account. If you are claiming Income Support, your Child Benefit will be deducted from your total allowance.

Your midwife, health visitor or Social Security office will be able to give you the necessary form.

Incapacity Benefit

If you can't get SMP or Maternity Allowance but you have worked and paid National Insurance in the last three years, you may be able to claim this benefit.

It is a weekly benefit paid from six weeks before the birth until two weeks after the birth. It is paid at a flat weekly rate of £46.15. You will need to check with Social Security office to see if you qualify.

Statutory Sick Pay

You will be disqualified from receiving Statutory Sick Pay (SSP) during the 18 weeks in which you are receiving SMP or MA. Your right to SSP returns at the end of the 18-week period.

If you take time off work due to illness you will normally be able to take sick leave and receive Statutory Sick Pay/Sickness Benefit up until the week of the baby's birth or until the week your Maternity Allowance is due to start. If, however, the illness is pregnancy-related and occurs after the beginning of the sixth week before the expected week of childbirth, entitlement to MA starts automatically and is payable from the first week in which the absence occurred or from the week after that, depending on whether the woman worked for her employer or was receiving SSP in the same week.

The Social Fund

If you or your partner are getting Income Support or Family Credit you may qualify for a Maternity Payment from the Social Fund in order to help you pay for things for your baby.

Maternity Rights and Benefits

The payment is £100 for each baby expected or born, but the total amount will be reduced by any savings of £500 or over which you, your partner or any dependent children who live with you may have. For every £1 of savings over £500 there will be a £1 deduction. Payment does not depend on National Insurance contributions.

You can apply any time from 11 weeks before your baby is due by asking your Social Security office for form SF100. You will need to send in your maternity certificate (Mat B1) with your application. If you do not have this yet you can send in a copy of your ante-natal clinic card instead. You can apply up until your baby is three months old. If you are applying after the birth, send a copy of the baby's birth certificate instead of the Mat B1.

Other Benefits
All pregnant women are entitled to the following:

Free NHS Dental Treatment. This applies during your pregnancy and for a year after your baby's birth. You can obtain more information from your local CHC, library, or Social Security office.

Free Prescriptions. You have the right to free prescriptions during pregnancy and for a year after your baby's birth. Your midwife, doctor or ante-natal clinic should have the appropriate forms for you to fill in.

In addition to the above benefits, women on a low income are also entitled to:

Free Milk and Vitamins. If you are receiving Income Support you are entitled to milk tokens which can be exchanged for 7 pints of cow's milk or powdered milk a week for yourself as well as for each of your children under five. For babies under one year old these tokens can be exchanged for powdered formula at your ante-natal clinic.

You are also entitled to free vitamins for yourself (while you are pregnant and breastfeeding) and for your children under five. These are available from your maternity or child health clinic. You will need to show your Income Support payment book or, if you are paid by giro, the letter which came with your giro.

Travelling Expenses. If you are getting Income Support or Family Credit (and sometimes if you are on a low income) you can claim your fares to and from hospital. Close relatives who are also on a low income may also be able to claim their fares when they visit you in hospital. Ask the midwives at your clinic, the hospital social worker, or the Social Security office for details.

Getting Back to Work

It is up to you when you return to work, provided that it is:

no later than the first working day after the end of your maternity leave period, *or*

within 28 weeks after the week in which the baby was born (for women who qualify for maternity absence), *or*

within any longer leave or absence period allowed on a voluntary or contractual basis by your employer.

When you resume work after statutory maternity leave you are entitled to have the same job and the same terms and conditions as if you had not been absent. If a redundancy situation arises during your maternity leave you should have been offered suitable alternative work at the time. You are also entitled to benefit from any general improvements to the rate of pay and other terms and conditions which may have been introduced for your grade or class of work while you were away.

Maternity Rights and Benefits

On returning to work after an additional maternity absence you are also entitled to have the same job and the same terms and conditions as if you had not been absent, unless a redundancy situation has arisen during the absence period or there is some other reason why it is not reasonably practicable for your employer to take you back in your original job (in which case you are generally entitled to be offered suitable alternative work). If your employer offers you suitable work and you unreasonably refuse, you may lose your right to a redundancy payment. If there is genuinely no suitable alternative work available, your maternity leave period and your maternity absence period should both count towards length of service in respect of redundancy payments.

You are generally entitled to benefit from any pay rises in your grade or class made during your absence. However, you may not necessarily be entitled to benefit from any improvements related to length of service (such as pension rights), nor does this period count towards assessing seniority. However, employers must at all times act lawfully under the Equal Pay Act 1970 and the Sex Discrimination Act 1975. So consult your union, Citizens Advice Bureau or the Maternity Alliance if you feel you have been unfairly treated or if you feel you are not benefiting from all the improvements you are entitled to.

If there is a reason other than redundancy which makes continuing in your present position unsuitable, your employer has a duty to find you suitable alternative employment. The terms and conditions of this job must be no less favourable to you than before, and the work should be both suitable and appropriate.

This is particularly relevant for women who work in environments which might not be conducive to the good health of a new and/or breastfeeding mother. Employers have a duty to protect the health and safety of all their employees including new and expectant mothers. All reasonable measures should be taken to prevent exposure to risks through removal of hazards or implementation of controls. Although they are not obliged to by law, employers should provide a safe and healthy environment for mothers to express and store breastmilk (toilets are not acceptable). New and expectant mothers must not be required to work at night if they have a medical certificate stating that the night work could damage their health or safety.

The ultimate action to avoid risk at work is to suspend a new or expectant mother on maternity grounds. If an employer exercises this option the mother must first be offered suitable alternative work. If none is available a woman on maternity suspension must be paid her normal wages or salary by her employer for as long as the suspension lasts. It is unlawful for an employer to dismiss an employee because of a health and safety regulation which could give rise to maternity suspension. All of these rights apply regardless of the employee's length of service or hours of work.

Once you return to work it is unlawful for your employer to dismiss you because you have taken advantage of your right to maternity leave and/or absence. If your employer refuses to let you return to work, then – subject to three exceptions – you can be regarded as having been unfairly dismissed and may take your employer to an Industrial Tribunal and make a claim of unfair dismissal.

The exceptions are that:

> you will not be considered dismissed if your original job is no longer available because of redundancy and there was no suitable alternative work which could be offered.

> you will not be regarded as unfairly dismissed if it was not reasonably practicable (on grounds other than redundancy) for you to be taken back in your original position and your employer has offered you suitable alternative employment which you either accepted or unreasonably refused, *or*

> it was not reasonably practicable for you to be taken back in your original job or to be offered suitable alternative employment and your employer (together with any

Maternity Rights and Benefits

associated employers) employed only five or fewer people at the point when your maternity leave period ended and your additional maternity absence period began.

The Juggling Act

Many women try to juggle work and home, only to end up exhausted and deeply depressed. Before you get to the point where dropping out altogether is the only option, consider other ways of working such as part-time work, job-sharing, flexible working hours, term-time working, career breaks, sabbaticals and working from home. The charity New Ways to Work (*see page 272 for address*) has pioneered in the field of changing cultural attitudes to work and finding solutions for individuals who cannot or do not wish to work in a traditional way. They can advise on the legal and practical aspects of options such as job-sharing.

At the moment employees have no statutory right to a job-share or part-time work. But under certain narrowly defined circumstances a female employee may be able to force an employer to allow her to job-share or work less than full-time. She will have to argue that she is being indirectly discriminated against under the Sex Discrimination Act 1975 by her employers' refusal to allow her to work part-time. It can be very difficult to bring a case of this nature to court, and even more difficult to win. However there have been some encouraging recent developments.

In March 1994 a landmark decision was made in the case *R v Secretary of State for Employment: ex parte EOC* which has gone some way towards clarifying women's legal position with regards to job protection. The House of Lords held that the Employment Protection (Consolidation) Act 1978 is discriminatory because it restricts the rights to claim unfair dismissal or a redundancy payment to employees who work at least eight hours a week, and imposes a longer service requirement (five years instead of two) on employees who work between eight and sixteen hours a week. Since 80 per cent of the UK's part-time workers are female, it was argued and upheld that these service qualifications are indirectly discriminatory because they disproportionately affect one sex more than the other.

Since then it has been accepted that, as long as a part-time employee has worked for the same employer for a continuous period of two years, she has the same rights to claim for unfair dismissal, redundancy pay and extended maternity leave as a full-time employee. This has been confirmed by succeeding cases of *Mediguard Services Ltd v Thame (1994)* and *Warren v Wylie and Wylie (1994) IRLR 316*, in which members of Industrial Tribunals accepted applicants' arguments for unfair dismissal on the basis of Article 119 of the Treaty of Rome, even where one applicant had worked less than eight hours a week.

At the moment, though, part-time employees have no right to overtime payments or Statutory Sick Pay. There is also no lower-earnings threshold, although all of these things are due for review in the European Court of Justice.

The British Government has consistently argued that improving conditions for part-time workers would make employers reluctant to create new part-time jobs and this, in turn, would disadvantage women. This has not, however, been the experience in the rest of Europe. Part-time employment is growing fastest in those European states with strong employment rights and benefits: Norway, Sweden, Denmark and the Netherlands.

When it comes to workplace crèches or nurseries, women often face the luck of the draw. Much depends on the size of the organization, their emphasis on personnel and whether or not they have a strong equal opportunities policy. Employers can be convinced to set up workplace nurseries, where none exist, provided they can be shown that it is both cost-effective and feasible within the structure of the organization. Working for Childcare (*see page 273 for address*) can help advise groups who wish to persuade their employers to set up a crèche or workplace nursery. They also publish a range of booklets which can enlighten employees and employers on the issues surrounding workplace childcare.

Maternity Rights and Benefits

Some unions can also be helpful. Invariably these are the ones which represent a large number of female workers. The banking union BIFU, UNISON (the Local Authority union), the General & Municipal Boilermakers (GMB), and the Transport and General (T&G) all have equality officers who can advise women on their options. The Trades Union Congress (TUC) has a strong equal opportunities policy and can supply a list of affiliated trade unions.

There is support around for women who want to exercise their rights to take paid leave, or to work in different ways. However, at the end of the day it is up to mothers to give voice to their needs and make sure they are heard and met. Supportive organizations can only help once mothers have taken the initiative to help themselves.

Sources:
Maternity Rights – A Guide for Employers and Employees (1995), Department of Trade and Industry
What Women Want, Lesley Abdela (The Body Shop)
Because of Her Sex, Kate Figes (Virago)

Appendix C
Support and Information

Lay and Voluntary Organizations

Action on Pre-Eclampsia
31–33 College Road
Harrow
Middlesex HA1 1EJ
(0181) 863–3271
Information and support for women with pre-eclampsia.

Active Birth Centre
25 Bickerton Road
London N19 5JT
(0171) 561–9006
Conducts a variety of classes and groups for mothers interested in active, physiological birth. Can put you in touch with local Active Birth teachers. Can supply pools for labour and birth.

Alcoholics Anonymous (AA)
AA General Service Office
PO Box 1
Stonebow House
Stonebow
York YO1 2NJ
(01904) 644 026
Network of independent self-help groups whose members encourage each other to keep off alcohol. Find your local group in the phone book or by contacting the General Service Office.

Association of Breastfeeding Mothers
26 Herschell Close
London SE26 4TH
(0181) 778-4769
Telephone advice and support groups for mothers who are breastfeeding or who wish to breastfeed.

Association for Improvements in the Maternity Services (AIMS)
40 Kingswood Avenue
London NW6 6LS
(0181) 865-5585
In Scotland:
40 Leamington Terrace
Edinburgh EH10 4JL
(0131) 229-6259
Support and information about parents' rights and choices, and advice about complaints procedures. Produces a quarterly journal covering current issues in maternity care.

Support and Information

Avon Episiotomy Support Group
PO Box 130
Weston-super-Mare
Avon BS23 4YJ
Self-help advice and a national network of support for women who have torn or had episiotomies. Please send SAE with enquiry.

BLISS
17-21 Emerald Street
London WC1N 3QL
(0171) 831-9393
Practical and emotional support for parents whose babies need intensive care or special support.

Caesarean Support Network
c/o Sheila Tunstall
2 Hurst Park Drive
Huyton
Liverpool L36 1TF
(0151) 480-1184
Emotional support and practical advice for women who have had or may need a caesarean delivery.

CRY-SIS
BM CRY-SIS
London WC1N 3XX
(0171) 404-5011
Support for parents of babies who cry excessively or those who have difficulty sleeping.

Gingerbread (England)
35 Wellington Street
London WC2E 7BB
(0171) 240-0953
Scotland: (0141) 353-0953
Northern Ireland: (01232) 231 417

Every Woman's BirthRights

Wales: (01792) 648 728
Self-help association for one-parent families. Local groups offer mutual support, information and advice.

Kith & Kids
404 Camden Road
London N7 0SJ
(0171) 700-2755
Advice and support for parents of disabled children.

La Leche League (Great Britain)
BM 3424
London WC1N 3XX
(0171) 242-1278 (24-hour answerphone)
Breastfeeding support and counselling for breastfeeding problems. Groups meet locally throughout the UK.

Meet-a-Mum Association (MAMA)
c/o Briony Hallam
58 Malden Avenue
South Norwood
London SE25 4HS
(0181) 656-7318
Support for mothers who feel lonely and isolated or are suffering from depression. Can put you in touch with other mothers in a similar situation and/or support groups.

Midwives Information and Resource Service (MIDIRS)
9 Elmdale Road
Clifton
Bristol BS8 1SL
(0117) 925-1791
Information service primarily for midwives, but non-members may also purchase copies of research papers concerned with maternity care.

Support and Information

Narcotics Anonymous
PO Box 417
London SW10 0DP
(0171) 498-9005
Self-help organization whose members help each other to stay off drugs. Write, or phone between 12 p.m. - 8 p.m., for advice and details of local groups.

National Childbirth Trust (NCT)
Alexandra House
Oldham Terrace
London W3 6NH
(0181) 992-8637
Information and support for all aspects of pregnancy and birth. Ante-natal classes and breastfeeding support. Local groups meet informally all over the country.

National Childminding Association
c/o Veronica Day
8 Masons Hill
Bromley
Kent BR2 9EY
(0181) 464-6164
Can supply a list of childminders in your area. Please send an A5 SAE on application.

National Council for One Parent Families
England, Northern Ireland and Wales:
255 Kentish Town Road
London NW5 2LX
(0171) 267-1361
Scotland: (0131) 556-3899
Information on benefits, rights in pregnancy, taxation, Social Security and maintenance.

National Information for Parents of Prematures – Education, Resources and Support (NIPPERS)
PO Box 1553
Wedmore
Somerset BS28 4LZ
(0171) 831-9393
Information and support for parents whose children have been born prematurely.

Pre-Eclamptic Toxaemia Society (PETS)
c/o Sharon Copping
Eaton Lodge
8 Southend Road
Hockley
Essex SS5 4QQ
(01702) 205 088
Support and information for women with pre-eclampsia. Has affiliated members worldwide. Please send SAE with enquiry.

Quit
102 Gloucester Place
London W1H 3DA
(0171) 487-3000 (helpline: 9.30 a.m. – 5.30 p.m.)
Advice on how to stop smoking, and details of local support services. Recorded message played outside office hours.

Relate: Marriage Guidance
Herbert Gray Cottage
Little Church Street
Rugby CV21 3AP
(01788) 573 241
Confidential counselling for relationship problems. Look in the phone book under 'Relate' for local branches.

Support and Information

Society to Support Home Confinements
'Lydgate'
Wolsingham
Bishop Auckland
Co Durham DL13 3HA
(01388) 528 044 (preferably after 6 p.m.)
Telephone support for women who are experiencing difficulties obtaining a home birth.

Splash Down Birth Pools
17 Wellington Terrace
Harrow-on-the-Hill
Middlesex HA1 3ER
(0181) 422-9308
Supplies birthing pools nationwide.

Stillbirth and Neonatal Death Society (SANDS)
28 Portland Place
London W1N 4DE
(0171) 436-5881
Information and a nationwide network of support groups for bereaved parents.

Support after Termination for Fetal Abnormality (SAFTA)
29 Soho Square
London W1V 6JB
(0171) 439-6124
Self-help charity. Support is given by parents who have had similar experiences.

Twins and Multiple Births Association (TAMBA)
PO Box 30
Little Sutton
South Wirral L66 1TH
(0151) 348-0020

Every Woman's BirthRights

Helpline: (01732) 868 000 (6 – 11 p.m. weekdays; 8 a.m. – 11 p.m. weekends)
Self-help organization to encourage and support parents of twins or more. Can advise on local support groups.

VBAC (Vaginal Birth After Caesarean) Information
c/o Gina Lowdon
Park View
Mill Corner
North Warnborough
Hook
Hampshire RG29 1HB
(01256) 704 871
Information and support for women who wish to avoid a repeat caesarean.

Government Bodies and Professional Organizations

Association of Radical Midwives
62 Greetby Hill
Ormskirk
Lancs L39 2DT
(01695) 572 776

Community Health Council
In Scotland, CHCs are called Local Health Councils; in Northern Ireland they are called Health and Social Services Councils.
Look in your phone book under your local health board.

District Health Authority
In Scotland: Health District; Northern Ireland: Health and Social Services District.
Look in your phone book under your local health board.

Support and Information

Family Health Services Authority (FHSA)
The address of your FHSA will be on your medical card and in the phone book. Can help you change doctors, and deals with complaints at the local level.

Independent Midwives Association
65 Mount Nod Road
London SW8 2LP
(0181) 677-9746
Can supply a list of independent midwives in your area experienced in home birth and advise if there is a birth centre near you.

National Board
Scotland: Scottish National Board, Northern Ireland: Northern Ireland National Board
Look in the phone book for the appropriate Board's number.

Regional Health Authority
In Scotland the RHA is known as the Health Board; Northern Ireland: Health and Social Services Board
Look in your phone book under your local health board.

Royal College of General Practitioners
14 Princes Gate
London SW7 1PU
(0171) 581-3232

Royal College of Midwives
15 Mansfield Street
London W1M 0BE
(0171) 580-6523

Royal College of Obstetricians and Gynaecologists
27 Sussex Place
London NW1 4RG
(0171) 262-5425

Every Woman's BirthRights

Complaints about Care

Action for Victims of Medical Accidents (AVMA)
Bank Chambers
1 London Road
Forest Hill
London SE23 3TP
(0181) 291-2793
Help and advice for parents who wish to take legal action.

Association for Improvements in the Maternity Services (AIMS)
Beverley Lawrence Beech (Hon Chair)
21 Iver Lane
Iver
Bucks SL0 9LH
(01753) 652 781

General Medical Council
44 Hallam Street
London W1N 6AE
(0171) 580-7642
Investigates complaints about the professional misconduct of doctors.

Health Information Service
(0800) 665 541
Freephone line for information about NHS services, including complaints procedures.

Ombudsman (Health Service Commissioner for England, Scotland and Wales)
Church House
Great Smith Street
London SW1P 3BW
(0171) 276-2035

Support and Information

Northern Ireland: (01232) 233 821
For complaints about the administrative aspects of care or the way a complaint has been handled.

Patients' Association
18 Victoria Square
London E2 9PF
(0181) 981-5676
Campaigns on behalf of NHS patients. Can give information and advice about making complaints.

United Kingdom Central Council (UKCC)
23 Portland Place
London W1M 3AF
(0171) 637-7181
Professional body which regulates and maintains the codes of conduct by which midwives, nurses and health visitors are bound.

Employment and Benefits

Advisory, Conciliation and Arbitration Service (ACAS)
Each region has its own branch of ACAS. Look in the phone book for your local branch. ACAS produces a range of booklets and leaflets on industrial relations and employment matters.

Benefits Agency
(0800) 666 555
Freephone advice line which can give you a good idea of any benefits for which you may qualify.

Citizens Advice Bureau
You will need to look in the phone book for the branch which serves your area.

Every Woman's BirthRights

Equal Opportunities Commission
Overseas House
Quay Street
Manchester M3 3HN
(0161) 833-9244
Can advise on women's rights in the workplace.

Law Centres Federation
Duchess House
18 Warren Street
London W1P 5DA
(0171) 387-8590
Maintains a register of local law centres.

Maternity Alliance
45 Beech Street
5th Floor
London EC2P 2LX
(0171) 588-8582
Information on all aspects of maternity services, rights at work, and benefits. Send an A5 SAE with requests for information.

New Ways to Work
309 Upper Street
London N1 2TY
(0171) 226-4026
An independent organization which promotes job-sharing and other flexible ways of working. Produces many useful publications.

Parents at Work
45 Beech Street
London EC2Y 8AB
(0171) 628-3578
Can advise on women's rights and options in the workplace.

Support and Information

Trades Union Congress (TUC)
Equal Rights Department
Great Russell Street
London WC1B 3LS
(0171) 636-4030
Can supply a list of affiliated trade unions. Unions can help bargain for equal pay, childcare, training for women, flexible working hours, career breaks and more.

Working for Childcare
727 Holloway Road
London N7 8JZ
(0171) 700-0281
Helps advise groups or individuals wishing to persuade an employer of the benefits of setting up a workplace nursery or crèche.

References

Introduction

1. Davis-Floyd, R. E. (1990), 'The Role of Obstetrical Rituals in the Resolution of Cultural Anomaly', *Social Science and Medicine* 31.2: 175–89. See also Rich, A. (1991), *Of Woman Born – Motherhood as Experience and Institution* (Virago)
2. Enkin, M., *et al.* (1995), *A Guide To Effective Care In Pregnancy and Childbirth* (2nd edn; Oxford University Press). Reviewed in Vines, G. (1995), 'Is there a database in the house?', *New Scientist* 21 January: 14–15
3. Northrup, C. (1995), *Women's Bodies, Women's Wisdom* (Piatkus)
4. Department of Health (1994), *Health and Personal Social Services Statistics for England 1994 Edition* (HMSO)

Chapter 1: Looking Ahead – Birth Options

1. Jackson, D. (1994), 'Choice – it depends on where you live', *AIMS Journal* 6.1: 11–12

2. Beech, B. A. L. (1991), *Who's Having Your Baby?* (Bedford Square Press)
3. Macfarlane, A. (1978), 'Variations in number of births and perinatal mortality by day of week in England and Wales', *BMJ* 2: 1670–73
4. Beech, B. A. L. (1991) *Who's Having Your Baby?* (Bedford Square Press)
5. Drife, J. (1994), 'Home Start for Mother', *Times* 26 April: 15
6. Report of the Clinical Studies Advisory Group (1995), *Women in Normal Labour* (HMSO)
7. Taylor, G. W. (1980), 'How safe is general practitioner obstetrics?', *Lancet* 2: 1287–89
8. Klein, M., *et al.* (1983), 'A comparison of low-risk pregnant women booked for delivery in two systems of care: shared-care (consultant) and integrated practice unit', *British Journal of Obstetrics and Gynaecology* 90: 118–22 and 123–28
9. Tew, M. (1986), 'Do obstetric intranatal interventions make birth safer?', *British Journal of Obstetrics and Gynaecology* 93: 659–74
10. Beech, B. A. L. (1991), *op cit*
11. Ford, C., Iliffe, S., Franklin, O. (1991), 'Outcome of planned home births in an inner city practice', *BMJ* 303: 1517–19
12. Demilew, J. (1994), 'Southeast London midwifery group practice', *MIDIRS Midwifery Digest* 4.3: 270–72
13. Report of the Expert Maternity Group (1994), *Changing Childbirth* (HMSO)
14. Campbell, R. (1984), 'Statistics and policy making in the maternity services' (lecture in symposium, Royal Society of Medicine) quoted in Kitzinger, S. (1987), *Freedom and Choice in Childbirth* (Penguin)
15. Tew, M. (1980), 'Is home a safer place?', *Health and Social Service Journal* 89: 702–705
16. Ford, C., *et al.* (1991), *op cit*
17. Gaskin, I. (1994), 'Statistics for 1888 births attended by the farm midwives, November 8, 1970 to April 1994', *The Birth Gazette* Summer Edition

References

18. Dodds, R., Newburn, M. (1995), *Availability of Home Birth – Experiences of women planning to give birth at home, and the responses of some General Practitioners* (NCT)
19. Report of the Expert Maternity Group (1993), *op cit*
20. Campbell, R., Macfarlane, A. (1990), 'Recent debate on the place of birth', in Garcia, J., Kilpatrick, R., Richards, M. (eds), *The Politics of Maternity Care* (Clarendon Press)
21. Royal College of Midwives News Release (1994), NR267/07/94
22. Buckley, R. (1995), 'How much of a problem are visitors on the labour suite?', *British Journal of Midwifery* 3.3: 168–70
23. Lewis, L. (1993), 'Who's knocking?', *Midwifery Matters* 58: 11–13
24. Flint, C. (1994), 'The woman now labouring on platform 12...', *MIDIRS Midwifery Digest* 4.3: 269
25. Simkin, P. (1993), 'When should a child attend a sibling's birth?', *Midwifery Today* 28: 37
26. Yates, P. (1990), *The Fun Starts Here* (Bloomsbury)
27. Gardosi, J., Sylvester S., B-Lynch, G. (1989), 'Alternative positions in the second stage of labour: a randomised trial', *British Journal of Obstetrics and Gynaecology* 96: 1290–96
28. Read, J. A., Miller, F. C., Paul, R. H. (1981), 'Ambulation versus oxytocin for labour enhancement', *American Journal of Obstetrics and Gynecology* 139: 669–72
29. Balaskas, J., Balaskas, A. (1988), *New Life* (Sidgwick & Jackson)
30. Enkin, M., *et al.* (1995) *A Guide to Effective Care in Pregnancy & Childbirth* (2nd edn; Oxford University Press)
31. Robertson, A. (1994), *Empowering Women* (Ace Graphics)
32. Enkin, M., *et al.* (1995), *op cit*
33. Balaskas J., Balaskas, A., *op cit*
34. Gestaldo, T. D. (1992), 'The significance of maternal position on pelvic outlet dimensions' (correspondence), *Birth* 19.4: 230
35. Crowley, P., *et al.* (1991), 'Delivery in an obstetric birth chair: a randomized controlled trial', *British Journal of Obstetrics and Gynaecology* 98: 667–74

36. Enkin, M., *et al.* (1995), *op cit*
37. Alderdice, F., *et al.* (1995) 'Labour and birth in water in England and Wales', *BMJ* 310: 837
38. Burns, F., Greenish, K. (1993), 'Pooling Information', *Nursing Times* 89.8: 47–49
39. Burke, E., Kilfoyle, A. (1995), 'A Cooperative Study of Waterbirth', *Midwives Chronicle* January: 3–7
40. *UKCC Position Statement on Water Births (1994)* (UKCC)
41. *Consent to Treatment* (1992), Medical Defence Union Ltd.
42. Hewson, B. (1993), 'Ethical triumph, or surgical rape?', *Solicitor's Journal* 26 Nov: 1182–83
43. Hewson, B. (1994), 'Court-ordered caesarean: ethical triumph or surgical rape?', *AIMS Journal* 6.2: 1–5
44. Royal College of Obstetricians and Gynaecologists (1994), 'A consideration of the law and ethics in relation to court-ordered obstetric intervention', *RCOG Guidelines – Ethics* (RCOG)

Chapter 2: Meeting the 'Experts'

1. Wagner, M. (1994), *Pursuing the Birth Machine – The Search for Appropriate Birth Technology* (Ace Graphics)
2. Roberts, H. (1985), *The Patient Patients – Women and Their Doctors* (Pandora)
3. Oakley, A. (1984), *The Captured Womb* (Blackwell)
4. Francombe, C., *et al.* (1993), *Caesarean Birth In Britain* (Middlesex University Press)
5. Klaus, M. H., *et al.* (1992), 'Maternal assistance and support in labour: father, nurse, midwife, or doula?', *Clinical Consultations in Obstetrics and Gynaecology* 4.4: 211–17
6. Sosa, R., *et al.* (1980), 'The effect of supportive companions on perinatal problems, length of labour and mother-infant interaction', *New England Journal of Medicine* 303: 597–600
7. Report of the Expert Maternity Group (1994), *Changing Childbirth* (HMSO)
8. Hundley, V. A., Cruickshank, F. M., *et al.* (1994), 'Midwife

managed delivery unit: a randomised controlled comparison with consultant led care', *BMJ* 309: 1400–1404
9. Paterson-Brown, S., Wyatt, J., Fisk, M. (1994), 'Are clinicians interested in up to date reviews of effective care?', *BMJ* 307: 1464
10. Vines, G. (1995), 'Is there a database in the house?', *New Scientist* 21 January: 14–15
11. Tew, M. (1990), *Safer Childbirth? – A Critical History of Maternity Care* (1st edn; Chapman & Hall)
12. Beech, B. A. L. (1995), '...And there's more from Leeds', *AIMS Journal* 7.1
13. Roberts, H. (1985), *op cit.*
14. Green, J., Kitzinger, J., Coupland, V. (1990), 'Stereotypes of childbearing women: a look at some evidence', *Midwifery* 6: 125–32
15. Green, J., Kitzinger, J., Coupland, V. (1989), 'Choice and control in childbirth', in *The Needs of Parents and Infants – Proceedings of a Symposium* (The Health Promotion Research Trust)

Chapter 3: The Ante-natal Routine

1. Tew, M. (1995), *Safer Childbirth? – A Critical History of Maternity Care* (Chapman & Hall)
2. Medical Officer of the Local Government Board (1915), *Memorandum on Health Visiting and on Maternity and Child Welfare Centres* (HMSO), quoted in Tew, M., (1995), *op cit*
3. Campion, S. (1950), *National Baby* (Ernest Benn)
4. Department of Health and Social Security: Central Health Services Council Standing Midwifery and Maternity Committee (1961), *Human Relations in Obstetrics* (HMSO), quoted in Tew, M., (1995) *op cit*
5. Office of Population Census and Survey (1994), Health and personal social services statistics for England (HMSO)
6. Kitzinger, S. (1984), *The Experience of Childbirth* (Penguin)
7. Office of Population Census and Survey (1990), *Mortality*

Statistics – Perinatal and Infant: Social and Biological Factors in England and Wales (HMSO)
8. Tew, M. (1995), *op cit*
9. Newnham, J., *et al.* (1993), 'Effects of frequent ultrasound during pregnancy: a randomised controlled trial', *Lancet* 342: 887–91
10. Enkin, M., (1995), *A Guide to Effective Care in Pregnancy and Childbirth* (Oxford University Press)
11. Meenan, A. L., Gaskin, I. M., Hunt, P., Ball, C. A. (1991), 'A new (old) maneuver for the management of shoulder dystocia', *The Journal of Family Practice* 32.6: 625–29
12. Hoffmeyer, G. J. (1991), 'External cephalic version at term: how high are the stakes?', *British Journal of Obstetrics and Gynaecology* 98: 1–3
13. Nwosu, E. C., Walkinshaw, S., *et al.* (1993), 'Undiagnosed breech', *British Journal of Obstetrics and Gynaecology* 100: 531–35
14. Enkin, M., *et al.* (1995), *op cit*
15. Wainer-Cohen, N. (1995), *Open Season – A Survival Guide for Natural Childbirth and VBAC in the 90s* (Bergin & Garvey)
16. Enkin, M., *et al.* (1995), *op cit*
17. Murphy, J., *et al.* (1986), 'Relation of haemoglobin levels in 1st and 2nd trimesters to outcome of pregnancy', *Lancet* 1: 992–94
18. Rasmussen, S., Oian, P. (1993), 'First and second trimester hemoglobin levels. Relation to birth weight and gestational age', *Acta Obstetrica Gynecologica Scandinavia* 72.4: 246–51
19. Barrett, J. F. R., *et al.* (1994), 'Absorption of non-haem iron from food during pregnancy', *BMJ* 309: 79–82
20. Enkin, M., *et al.* (1995), *op cit*
21. Enkin, M., *et al.* (1995), *ibid*
22. Saari-Kemppainen, A., *et al.* (1990), 'Ultrasound screening and perinatal mortality: controlled trial of systematic one-stage screening in pregnancy', *Lancet* 336: 387–91
23. Health Education Authority (1993), *Smoking and Pregnancy – Tracking Study* (HEA)

References

24. Whent, H. (1994), *Smoking and Pregnancy – A guide for Purchasers and Providers* (HEA)
25. Madeley, R. J., *et al.* (1989), 'Nottingham mothers stop smoking project – survey of smoking in pregnancy', *Community Medicine* 11.2: 124–30
26. Frank, P., *et al.* (1994), 'Effect of change in maternal smoking habits in early pregnancy on infant birthweight', *British Journal of General Practice* 44: 57–59
27. Mitchell, E. A., *et al.* (1993), 'Smoking and the sudden infant death syndrome', *Pediatrics* 91.5: 893–96
28. Hansen J. W., *et al.* (1978), 'Effects of moderate alcohol consumption during pregnancy on fetal growth and morphogenesis', *Journal of Pediatrics* 92.3: 457–60
29. Plant, M. L. (1984), 'Drinking amongst pregnant women: some initial results from a prospective study', *Alcohol Alcohol* 19.2: 153–57
30. Scott, E., Anderson, P. (1990), 'Randomised controlled trial of general practitioner intervention in patients with excessive alcohol consumption', *Drugs and Alcohol Review* 10: 313–21
31. Enkin, M., *et al.* (1995), *op cit*
32. Balaskas, J. (1990), *Natural Pregnancy* (Sidgwick & Jackson)
33. Odent, M. (1993), 'Midwives are better than electronics', *Caduceus* 20: 11–13
34. Odent, M. (1994), *Birth Reborn* (2nd edn; Souvenir Press)
35. Green, M., Kitzinger, J., Coupland, V. (1990), 'Stereotypes of childbearing women: a look at some evidence', *Midwifery* 6: 125–32
36. Francis, H. (1995), 'Obstetrics: a consumer oriented service? The case against', *Maternal and Child Health* 10.3: 69–72
37. McParland, P., Johnson, H. (1993), 'Time to reinvent the wheel', *British Journal of Obstetrics and Gynaecology* 100: 1061–62
38. Rowlands, S., Royston, P. (1993), 'Estimated date of delivery from last menstrual period and ultrasound scan: which is more accurate?', *British Journal of General Practice* 43: 322–25

39. Saunders, N., Paterson, C. (1991), 'Can we abandon Naegle's rule?', *Lancet* 337: 600–601
40. Yoong, A., *et al.* (1993), 'Medical audit: the problem of missing case notes', *Health Trends* 25: 114–16
41. Lovell, A., *et al.* (1987), 'The St Thomas's Hospital maternity case notes study: a randomised controlled trial to assess the effects of giving expectant mothers their own maternity case notes', *Paediatric and Perinatal Epidemiology* 1.1: 57–66
42. Hewison, A. (1993), 'The language of labour: an examination of the discourses of childbirth', *Midwifery* 9: 225–34
43. Robertson, A. (1994), *Empowering Women – Teaching Active Birth in the 90s* (Ace Graphics)
44. Tannen, D. (1991), *You Just Don't Understand – Women and Men in Conversation* (Virago)
45. Shapiro, M. C., *et al.* (1993), 'Information control and the exercise of power in the obstetrical encounter', *Social Science in Medicine* 17.3: 139–46

Chapter 4: Testing, Testing

1. Editorial (1984), 'Diagnostic ultrasound in pregnancy', *Lancet* 28 July: 201–202
2. Ewigman, B. G., *et al.* (1993), 'Effects of prenatal ultrasound screening on perinatal outcome', *New England Journal of Medicine* 329.12: 821–27
3. Saari-Kemppainen, A., *et al.* (1990), 'Ultrasound screening and perinatal mortality: controlled trial of systematic one-stage screening in pregnancy', *Lancet* 336: 387–91
4. Lorenz, R. P. (1990), 'Randomized prospective trial comparing ultrasonography and pelvic examination for preterm labor surveillance', *American Journal of Obstetrics and Gynecology* 162: 1603–10
5. Newnham, J. P., *et al.* (1993), 'Effects of frequent ultrasound during pregnancy: a randomised controlled trial', *Lancet* 342: 887–91

References

6. Thacker, S. (1985), 'Quality of controlled clinical trials. The case of imaging ultrasound in obstetrics: a review', *British Journal of Obstetrics and Gynaecology* 92: 437–44
7. Bosward, K. L., et al. (1993), 'Heating of guinea-pig fetal brain during exposure to pulsed ultrasound', *Ultrasound in Medicine and Biology* 19.5: 415–24
8. Mole, R. (1986), 'Possible hazards of imaging and Doppler ultrasound in obstetrics', *Birth* 13: 29–37
9. Salvesen, K. A., et al. (1993), 'Routine ultrasonography in utero and subsequent handedness and neurological development', *Lancet* 307: 159–64
10. Stark, et al. (1984), 'Short- and long-term risks after exposure to diagnostic ultrasound in utero', *Obstetrics and Gynecology* 63: 194–200
11. Campbell, J. D., et al. (1993), 'Case-control study of prenatal ultrasonography in children with delayed speech', *Canadian Medical Association Journal* 149.10: 1435–40
12. Beech, B. A. L., Robinson, J. (1994), *Ultrasound? Unsound* (AIMS)
13. Robinson, J. (1994), 'What really happened in Cardiff?', *AIMS Journal* 6.4: 9–10
14. Rogers, L. (1995) 'Doubts over pregnancy scans as doctors abort healthy babies', *Sunday Times* 15 October: 1
15. Enkin, M., et al. (1990), *A Guide to Effective Care in Pregnancy and Childbirth* (1st edn; Oxford University Press)
16. Hammond, P. (1994), 'Test pest', *Nursing Times* 90.32: 60
17. Robinson, L., Grau, P., Crandall, B. F. (1989), 'Pregnancy outcomes after increasing maternal serum alphafetoprotein levels', *Obstetrics and Gynecology* 74: 17–20
18. Cashner, K. A., et al. (1987), 'Spontaneous fetal loss after demonstration of a live fetus in the first trimester', *Obstetrics and Gynecology* 70: 827–30
19. Lin, S., et al. (1994), 'Pregnancy outcome following early versus traditional amniocentesis: A single institution case controlled study', *American Journal of Obstetrics and Gynecology* 170: 272

20. Haddow, J. E., *et al.* (1994), 'Reducing the need for amniocentesis in women 35 years of age or older with serum markers for screening', *New England Journal of Medicine* 330.16: 1114–18
21. Alberman, E., Dennis, K. J. (1984), 'Late abortions in England and Wales – Report of a national confidential study' (Royal College of Obstetricians and Gynaecologists). See also Hibbard, B. N., *et al.* (1985), 'Can we afford screening for neural tube defects? The South Wales experience', *BMJ* 290: 293–95
22. Medical Research Council European Trial of Chorionic Villus Sampling (1991), *Lancet* 337: 1491–99
23. Brambati, B., *et al.* (1987), 'Transabdominal chorionic villus sampling: a freehand ultrasound-guided technique', *American Journal of Obstetrics and Gynecology* 157: 134–37
24. Blakemore K. J., *et al.* (1986), 'Rise in maternal serum alphafetoprotein concentration after chorionic villus sampling and the possibility of isoimmunization', *American Journal of Obstetrics and Gynecology* 155: 988–93
25. Firth, H. V., *et al.* (1994), 'Analysis of limb reduction defects in babies exposed to chorionic villus sampling', *Lancet* 343: 1069–71
26. Firth, H., Boyd, P., *et al.* (1991), 'Severe limb abnormalities after chorionic villus sampling at 55–66 days' gestation', *Lancet* 337: 762–63
27. Robinson, G. E., *et al.* (1991), 'Psychological reactions to pregnancy loss after prenatal diagnostic testing: preliminary results', *Journal of Psychosomatic Obstetrics & Gynaecology* 12: 181–92
28. Balaskas, J., Balaskas, A. (1988), *New Life* (Sidgwick & Jackson)
29. Thubisi, M., *et al.* (1993), 'Vaginal delivery after previous caesarean section: is pelvimetry a reliable predictor?', *British Journal of Obstetrics and Gynaecology* 100: 421–24
30. Flint, C. (1986), *Sensitive Midwifery* (Butterworth Heinemann)

References

Chapter 5: Managing Labour

1. Kierse, M. J. N. C. (1993), 'A final comment ... managing the uterus, the woman, or whom?', *Birth* 20.3: 150-61
2. Gaskin, I. M. (1978), *Spiritual Midwifery* (The Book Publishing Company)
3. Arms, S. (1975), *Immaculate Deception: A New Look At Women and Childbirth in America* (Houghton Mifflin)
4. National Childbirth Trust (1989), *Rupture of the Membranes in Labour* (NCT)
5. Wagner, M. (1994), *Pursuing the Birth Machine – The Search for Appropriate Birth Technology* (Ace Graphics)
6. Tew, M. (1986), 'Do obstetric intranatal interventions make birth safer?', *British Journal of Obstetrics and Gynaecology* 93: 659-74
7. Cardozo, L. (1993), 'Is routine induction of labour at term ever justified?', *BMJ* 306: 840-41
8. Thornton, J. G., Lilford, R. J. (1994), 'Active management of labour: current knowledge and research issues', *BMJ* 309: 366-69
9. Gibbs, D. M. F., Cardozo, L. D., *et al.* (1982), 'Prolonged pregnancy: is induction of labour indicated?', *British Journal of Obstetrics and Gynaecology* 89: 292-95
10. Alfirevic, Z., Walkinshaw, S. A. (1994), 'Management of post-term pregnancy – to induce or not?', *British Journal of Hospital Medicine* 52.5: 218-21
11. Tew, M. (1986), *op cit*
12. Olah, K. S. J., Neilson, J. P. (1994), 'Failure to progress in the management of labour', *British Journal of Obstetrics and Gynaecology* 101: 1-3
13. Thornton, J. G., Lilford, R. J. (1994), *op cit*
14. Garcia, J., Garforth, S. (1989), 'Labour and delivery routines in English consultant maternity units', *Midwifery* 5: 155-62
15. Enkin, M., *et al.* (1995), *A Guide to Effective Care in Pregnancy & Childbirth* (2nd edn; Oxford University Press)

16. Molloy, B. G., et al. (1987), 'Delivery after caesarean section: review of 2,176 consecutive cases', *BMJ* 294: 1645–46
17. Enkin, M., et al. (1991), *A Guide to Effective Care in Pregnancy & Childbirth* (1st edn; Oxford University Press)
18. Alott, H. A., Palmer, C. R. (1993), 'Sweeping the membranes: a valid procedure in stimulating the onset of labour?', *British Journal of Obstetrics and Gynaecology* 100: 898–903
19. Simkin, P. (1986), 'Is Anyone Listening? The Lack of Clinical Impact of Randomized Controlled Trial of Electronic Fetal Monitoring', *Birth* 13.4: 219–20
20. Neilson, J. P. (1994), 'Electronic fetal heart rate monitoring during labour: information from randomized trials', *Birth* 21.2: 101–104
21. MacDonald, D., et al. (1985), 'The Dublin randomized controlled trial of intrapartum fetal heart rate monitoring', *American Journal of Obstetrics and Gynecology* 152: 524–39
22. Wagner, M. (1994), *op cit*
23. Green, J. M. (1993), 'Expectations and experiences of pain in labor: findings from a large prospective study', *Birth* 20.2: 65–72
24. Jacobson, B., Nyberg, K., et al. (1990), 'Opiate addiction in adult offspring through possible imprinting after obstetric treatment', *BMJ* 301: 1067–70. Also Jacobson, B., Nyberg, K. (1988), 'Obstetric pain medication and eventual adult amphetamine addiction in offspring', *Acta Obstetrica Gynaecologica Scandinavia* 67: 677–82
25. Chamberlain, G., et al. (1993), *Pain and its Relief in Childbirth* (Churchill Livingstone)
26. *Ibid*
27. Howell, C., Chalmers, I. (1992), 'A review of prospectively controlled comparisons of epidural with non-epidural forms of pain relief during labor', *International Journal of Obstetric Anaesthesia* 1: 93–110
28. Maccaulay, J. H., et al. (1992), 'Epidural analgesia in labour and fetal hyperthermia', *Obstetrics and Gynecology* 80.4: 665–69

References

29. Cartwright, A. (1979), *The Diagnosis of Labour* (Tavistock), quoted in Wagner, M. (1994), *op cit*
30. MacArthur, C., Lewis, M., Knox, E. G. (1992), 'Investigation of long-term problems after obstetric epidural anaesthesia', *BMJ* 304: 1279–82
31. Haire, D. (1994) 'Obstetric drugs and procedures: their effects on mother and baby (Part 1)', *AIMS (Australia) Quarterly Journal* 6.1: 1–8
32. Thorp, J. A., *et al.* (1993), 'The effect of intrapartum epidural analgesia on nulliparous labour: a randomized, controlled, retrospective trial', *American Journal of Obstetrics and Gynecology* 169: 851–58
33. Haire, D. (1994), *op cit*
34. Wagner, M. (1994), *op cit*
35. Tew, M. (1995), *Safer Childbirth? – A Critical History of Maternity Care* (Chapman & Hall)
36. Kitzinger, S., Simkin, P. (1986), *Episiotomy and the Second Stage of Labour* (Pennypress)
37. Rajkhowa, M. (1994), 'Forceps or ventouse?', *Maternal and Child Health* 19.8: 248–50, 252
38. Johanson, R., *et al.* (1993), 'Health after childbirth; a comparison of normal and assisted vaginal delivery', *Midwifery* 9: 161–68
39. Rajkhowa, M., *et al.* (1994), *op cit*
40. Francombe, C., *et al.* (1994), *Caesarean Birth in Britain* (1994 Supplement; NCT & Middlesex University Press)
41. O'Driscoll, K., Foley, M. (1983), 'Correlation of decrease in perinatal mortality and increase of caesarean section rates', *Obstetrics and Gynecology* 61: 1–5
42. Enkin, M., *et al.* (1995) *op cit*
43. Hillan, E. M. (1992), 'Short-term morbidity associated with caesarean delivery', *Birth* 19.4: 190–94
44. Hewson, B. (1993), 'Total cost of caesarean births in UK is unnecessarily high' (correspondence), *Financial Times* 17 September

45. Francombe, C., *et al.* (1993), *Caesarean Birth in Britain* (Middlesex University Press)
46. Rubin, G., Peterson, H. B., Rochat, R. W., *et al.* (1981), 'Maternal death after caesarean section in Georgia', *American Journal of Obstetrics and Gynecology* 139: 681–85
47. Wainer-Cohen, N., Edner, L. J. (1983), *Silent Knife – Caesarean Prevention and Vaginal Birth After Caesarean* (Bergin & Garvey)
48. Flint, C. (1986), *Sensitive Midwifery* (Butterworth Heinemann)
49. Enkin, M. (1995), *op cit*
50. Lavin, J., *et al.* (1982), 'Vaginal delivery in patients with a prior caesarean section', *Obstetrics and Gynecology* 59: 135
51. Francombe, C., *et al.* (1993), *op cit*
52. *Ibid*
53. *Ibid*
54. Beech, B. A. L., (1995), 'Conscious during a general anaesthetic caesarean operation', *AIMS Journal* 7.3: 8–10
55. Atiba, E. O., *et al.* (1993), 'Patient's expectation and caesarean section rate', *The Lancet* 341: 246
56. Lagercrantz, H., Slotkin, T. A. (1986), 'The "stress" of being born', *Scientific Arena* April: 92–102
57. Molloy, B. G., Sheil, O., Duignan, N. M. (1987), 'Delivery after caesarean section: review of 2176 consecutive cases', *BMJ* 294: 1645–47
58. Inch, S. (1983), 'Management of the third stage of labor – another cascade of intervention?', *Midwifery* 1: 114–22
59. Edwards, N. P. (1995), *Delivering Your Placenta – The Third Stage*, (AIMS)
60. Inch, S. (1983), *op cit*
61. Edwards, N. P. (1995), *op cit*

Chapter 6: Back to Normal?

1. Kitzinger, S. (1975), 'The fourth trimester?', *Midwife, Health Visitor & Community Nurse* 11: 118–21

References

2. Elliott, S. A. (1990), Commentary on 'Childbirth as a Life Event', *Journal of Reproductive and Infant Psychology* 8.2: 147–59
3. Lareya, M. (1989), 'Midwives' and mothers' perceptions of motherhood', in Robinson, S., Thompson, A. (eds), *Midwives, Research and Childbirth, 1* (Chapman & Hall)
4. Simkin, P. (1991), 'Just another day in a woman's life? Women's long-term perceptions of their first birth experience, Part 1', *Birth* 18.4: 203–10; also Simkin, P. (1992), 'Just another day in a woman's life? Women's long-term perceptions of their first birth experience, Part 2', *Birth* 19.2: 64–81
5. Hall, M. H. *et al.* (1989), 'Mode of delivery and future fertility', *British Journal of Obstetrics and Gynaecology* 96: 1297–1303
6. Johanson, R., Wilkinson, P., *et al.* (1993), 'Health after childbirth: a comparison of normal and assisted vaginal delivery', *Midwifery* 9: 161–68
7. Trevelyan, J. (1994), 'Bad tidings of great joy', *The Guardian* 21 June: 19
8. MacArthur, C., *et al.* (1991), *Health After Childbirth* (HMSO)
9. MacArthur, C., Lewis, M., Knox, E. G. (1991), 'Health after Childbirth', *British Journal of Obstetrics and Gynaecology* 98: 1193–95
10. Thune-Larsen, K. B., Moller-Pedersen, K. (1988), 'Childbirth Experience and Postpartum Emotional Disturbance', *Journal of Reproductive and Infant Psychology* 6.4: 229–40
11. Jones, C. (1991), 'Beating the Baby Blues', *Special Delivery* Winter edition: 12
12. Maclean, G. D. (1994), 'Safe motherhood in the United Kingdom', *Modern Midwife* 4.6: 10–14
13. Burgess, V., Ripley, E., Hilton, T. (1987), 'Sex after Childbirth', *Mother* October: 6–9
14. Victor, C., Barrett, G. and the National Childbirth Trust (1994), 'Is there sex after childbirth?', *New Generation* June: 24–25
15. Glazener, C. M., Abdalla, M., *et al.* (1995), 'Postnatal maternal morbidity: extent, causes: prevention and treatment', *British Journal of Obstetrics and Gynaecology* 102: 282–87

16. Sleep, J., Grant, A. (1987), 'West Berkshire perineal management trial: three year follow-up', *BMJ* 295: 749–51
17. Glazener, C. M. A., Abdalla, M. I., Russell, I. T., Templeton, A. (1993), 'Postnatal care – a survey of patient experiences', *British Journal of Midwifery* 1: 67–77
18. Priya, J. V. (1992), *Birth Traditions & Modern Pregnancy Care* (Element)
19. Eisenberg, A., Murkoff, H. E., Hathaway, S. E. (1990), *What to Expect When You're Expecting* (Piatkus)

Appendix A

1. Beech, B. A. L. (1991), *Who's Having Your Baby?* (Bedford Square Press)
2. Hickson, G., *et al.* (1994), 'Obstetricians' prior mal-practice experience and patients' satisfaction with care', *Journal of the American Medical Association* 272: 1583–87
3. Beech, B. A. L. (1991), *op cit*

Index

abdominal belt monitor 179, 182–4
abdominal palpation 131
abnormality 20, 82–4, 79, 126, 133, 138, 157–9
  result of CVS 153
  result of ultrasound 137
abortion
  of female fetuses 116
  for fetal abnormality 79
  of normal fetuses 138, 150
  see also termination
acceleration of labour see augmentation of labour
access to Health Records Act 1990 117, 236
Active Birth Movement 109, 164
active management 161–4, 167
acupressure 91
acupuncture
  for breech position 91
  to start labour 168
AIDS 128
alcohol 78, 80, 103–5

allergic reaction
  to opiates 192
alphafetoprotein (AFP)
  testing 141–5, 147, 150
  levels in mother's blood 143
amniocentesis 144, 146–52, 154, 159
  revealing sex of baby 116
amniotomy see artificial rupture of membranes (ARM)
anaemia 80, 97–9, 221
anaesthetic 187, 188, 204
  failure during caesarean 214
  failed epidural 195
  see also epidural, general anaesthetic
analgesic 187, 188
anencephaly 83, 143, 159
ante-natal care 59, 77–81
  effectiveness of 79, 82
  failure of 233
  home birth 18
  during Second World War 79

ante-natal classes 80, 108–11, 231, 233
  time-off for 244
ante-natal testing 126, 157–9
  see also individual tests
anti-D immunisation 128
APGAR score 7, 82, 117, 137, 165, 182, 192
Arms, Suzanne 163
artificial rupture of membranes (ARM) 165, 168, 169–71, 175, 178, 184, 202
assisting labour 201–18
  see also caesarean, forceps, gravity, walking, ventouse
Association for Improvements in the Maternity Services (AIMS) 9, 20, 97, 236, 241
Association for Victims of Medical Accidents 241
Association of Radical Midwives 55

291

augmentation of labour 7, 28, 31, 167, 202, 208
  see also individual methods

baby
  testing blood sugar 100
  role in labour 40, 164
  sex of 116
  well-being 82–92
backache
  caused by epidural 196, 228
  in labour 88
Balaskas, Janet 31, 164
bed rest
  mothers with twins 88
  for pre-eclampsia 94
Beech, Beverley Lawrence 9, 240
birth
  alone 25
  depression after 228–30
  as a life event 224
  positions for 28–34
  wider perspective 2
birth centres 10
birth chair/bed 32–4
birth companions
  adults 22–5
  children 25–8
birth plans 111–14
birth stool 32, 168
birth wheel 32
birthweight
  and CVS 153
  and home birth 20
  predictions about 85–6
  and smoking 101
  and twins 88
'blind amniocentesis' 148
blood
  composition during pregnancy 97
blood sugar
  levels in pregnancy 14, 99
blood tests 39, 127–8, 142–6, 157

breaking the waters see artificial rupture of membranes
breastfeeding 16, 114, 216
breech position 71, 88–91
  and caesarean 211,
  and VBAC 213
Brewer, Tom 95
bupivacaine 193, 197

caesarean 4, 11, 16, 111, 116, 161, 171, 192, 201, 205, 207, 209–18, 231
  for breech baby 90
  elective 214–15
  enforced 39
  resulting from epidural 198
  feelings after 212
  for HIV positive mothers 211
  monitoring leading to 183
  for pre-eclampsia 96
  and pre-term birth 117
  and secondary infertility 225
Campbell and Macfarlane 21
cardiotocographic monitoring (CTG) 182
cardiovascular malformations 83
case notes 117–20, 236
caster oil 168
catecholamines 215
central nervous system malformations 83
cephalopelvic disproportion 156, 210
cerivicograms 164
cervix 40, 41, 121, 149, 152, 161, 162, 164, 167, 168, 169, 171, 175, 176, 215
Changing Childbirth 17
changing practitioners 49
child benefit 251
chorionic villi 153
chorionic villus sampling (CVS) 147, 152–5, 159
cleft lip/palate 83

club foot 83
coccyx 30
Cochrane Collaboration
  Pregnancy & Childbirth Database 61
Community Health Council (CHC) 2, 4, 63, 236, 239
complaining about care 235–42
consultant see obstetrician
consultant unit see hospital
consumers
  women as xiii, 6, 44
continuity of care 51, 165
continuous monitoring 181–6
  see also under individual methods of monitoring
contractions 28, 29, 30, 162, 165, 167, 168, 171–2, 183, 190, 196, 203, 206
  after amniocentesis 148
controlled cord traction (CCT) 219
cord clamping 219
cord prolapse 170, 213
cordocentesis 157
counselling
  genetic 149, 150

Data Protection Act 1987 119, 236
death see mortality
depression
  after birth 80, 225, 228–30
dextrose see glucose
diabetes
  in mothers 86, 93
'diagnostic rape' 136
diagnostic tests 126, 146–57
  see also specific tests
diamorphene 191–2
diet 78
  and pre-eclampsia 95
  in pregnancy 105–8
  see also food
disclaimers
  for home birth 18

Index

for hospital birth 15
for water birth 38
diuretics 96
domino scheme 2, 10, 11–12, 55
doppler 132, 137, 180
doula 53
Down's Syndrome 83, 127, 135, 141, 142, 143, 147, 149
drugs
  effect on baby 188–9
  in labour 28, 41
dystocia
  shoulder 87, 168, 215

eclampsia 79, 93
elective caesarean 214–15
electronic fetal monitoring (EFM) 78, 109, 169, 173, 178, 182, 195,
  caesareans caused by 210
endorphins 172, 178, 187
entenox 59, 190
epidural 7, 96, 109, 178, 187, 193–200, 206, 214, 227
  failed 194
  mobile 196, 198
  side effects 195–7
episiotomy 4, 33, 72, 187, 201–5, 227, 231
ergometrine 220
estimated delivery date (EDD) 114–16, 166
  usefulness of ultrasound 85
external version 89–90, 91
'extra contractual referral' 5

'failure to progress' 161, 164, 166, 167, 210, 213
false positive/negative 126, 142
Family Health Services Authority 50, 52, 238
Farm, The 21
fetal alcohol syndrome 105
fetal blood sampling 184
  see also cordocentesis

fetal distress 7, 178, 179
  resulting in caesarean 210, 213
  caused by epidural 196
  caused by induction 172
  caused by lying down in labour 191
'fetal extraction' 205
fetal growth
  abdominal palpation 131
  measuring fundal height 139
  relation to mother's weight 130
fetal heart monitor 132
fetal position 88–92
fetomaternal haemorrhage 153
fetus 121
  positions during pregnancy 88–92
  standing in law 39
  viable 115
Flint, Caroline 24, 158, 212
flying squad 19
food
  in labour 13–14
forceps 4, 7, 8, 109, 171, 201, 202, 205–9, 227, 231
  cause of post-natal pain 226
'fourth trimester' 224

gas & air see Entenox
Gaskin, Ina May 162
general anaesthetic 192–3, 211
  and denial of food 13, 96
General Medical Council 239
genetic counselling 149
German measles see Rubella
gestational diabetes 99–100
glucose drip 13, 216
  harm to baby 14
GP unit 2, 6–8, 48
GPs 5, 8, 10, 15, 16, 17, 19, 43, 48, 49–52, 53, 63, 68, 115, 127, 135, 227
  complaints about 238

gravity
  as aid to labour 28, 198, 202
growth charts 85
growth retardation 85–6, 133
  caused by alcohol, 105
  resulting from dietary restriction 107
  inductions for 166–7
  caused by pre-eclampsia 93, 96
  caused by smoking 103

haemorrhoids 33, 228
health
  after birth 225
health visitors 43, 65–7, 68, 229
  complaints about 239
healthcare policies 44
heroin see diamorphene
Hewson, Barbara 39
high blood pressure
  drugs for 96
  with pre-eclampsia 93
  smoking 103
  'white coat hypertension' 130
Hippocratic Oath 62
histology 150
HIV testing 128
  and caesarean delivery 211
home birth 1, 15–22, 24, 29, 48, 52, 62, 230
home from home units see GP units
hospitals 1, 3–10, 23, 29, 34, 35, 47, 54, 55, 62, 109, 138, 139, 230
  complaining about care 238
  food in 13–14
  leaving 10–13
hydrocephalus 83
hydrospadies 83
hypertension see high blood pressure

293

hyperthermia
  in baby during waterbirth 36
  caused by epidural 195–6
hypoglycaemia
  in baby 14, 100
hypoxia 167

idopathic respiratory distress 220
in vitro fertilisation (IVF) 87
incapacity benefit 252
incontinence 228
independent midwives 2, 58–60
  and home birth 17
  insurance for 2, 59
Independent Midwives Association (IMA) 10, 59
induction 4, 7, 8, 10, 164–77
  failed 173
  for growth retardation 85
  in private hospitals 10
  see also individual methods
information
  mother's difficulty in getting 119, 123
intermittent monitoring 179–81
  see also individual methods of monitoring
interventions 3–4, 8, 47, 53, 64, 225
  need for monitoring during 178
  in post-natal period 233
  reduced by labour in water 35, 37
iron 97, 98

Jackson, Deborah, 2
jaundice
  caused by over-transfusion 221
  caused by syntocinon 173
job
  changing 244
  losing 245

'jumping babies' 137

ketones 14, 129
kick chart 86
Kith and Kids 84
Kitzinger, Sheila 83
kneeling position 173

labour
  active management of 161–4
  assisting 201–18
  baby's role in 40
  days of the week 4
  gravity as an aid 28
  media images of 29
  'normal' 3, 6
  positions for 28–34
  privacy during 15, 23–24
  prolonged by epidural 198
  see also caesarean, forceps, gravity, walking, ventouse
  slow see dystocia
lateral position 31
law
  baby's right to treatment 39
  baby's sex 116
  birth partners 24–5
  consent to treatment 48
  enforced caesarean 39–40
  home birth 15
  attending ultrasound scans 139
legal action
  doctors fear of 46, 116, 210
  taking 240
lifestyle 101–8
'light for dates' 85
limb deformities
  caused by CVS 153
lithotomy position 30
low blood pressure
  effect of heroin 192
  with epidural 196
  and water birth 35
lovemaking
  to stimulate labour 168

maternity absence 248–9
maternity allowance 251
maternity care
  harmful procedures xii
maternity leave 245–8
maternity rights and benefits 243–59
  see also benefits
mecomium 169
Medical Defence Union 39
medical education 47, 74, 233
medical language 73, 108, 121–4
Medical Research Council 152
'medicalese' 108
midwifery unit see GP unit
midwives xiv, xv, 8, 11, 15, 16, 18, 19, 22, 23, 29, 35, 37, 38, 43, 45, 52, 53–60, 63, 73, 74, 106, 115, 117, 135, 164, 178, 196, 224
  complaints about 239
miscarriage
  after amniocentesis 145, 147, 149, 154
  after CVS 154
  and smoking 102
mobility
  loss of in labour 179, 182, 196
monitoring 4, 177–86
  lack of mobility 173, 179
  see also individual methods of monitoring
mortality
  and caesarean 211
  impact of caesarean 209
  from CVS 152
  home birth 20
  effect of inductions 165
  infant 8, 21, 79, 85
  mother 77, 79, 193
  effect of smoking 101
  waterbirth 36
mother's well-being 92–100
mothers
  consent to treatment 39, 48
  as consumers xii, xiii, 6, 48
  and doctors 45–9

Index

as good patients 74
in hospital power structure 45
multiple pregnancy 78, 87-8, 143, 221

naloxone 191
NCT 4, 20, 21, 75, 88, 97, 109, 165
neck and shoulder pain 193, 228
neural tube defects 141, 143, 147, 150
nipple stimulation
aid to labour 168, 221
Northrup, Christiane xiii
nuchal scan 135-6, 149

obstetric wheels 115
obstetricians 15, 18, 34, 36, 40, 43, 45, 60-65, 69, 72, 164, 196
complaints about 239
epidurals and job satisfaction 196
in private hospitals 9
obstetrics list 50, 51
Odent, Michel 24, 109, 110
oedema
and inductions 173
and pre-eclampsia 92, 95
ombudsman 238, 241
overdue *see* post-mature pregnancy
oxytocin 29, 162

paediatricians 43, 67-9
pain 28, 97, 186-90
after birth 226-8
pain relief 16, 30, 35, 190-200
after a caesarean 215
best time to use drugs 188
from upright positions 31
from walking 28
from water 37
'parentcraft classes' 109
partograms 164
Patient's Charter 70

pelvic floor exercises 231
pelvimetry 155-7
pelvis
in labour 30, 31, 40, 90, 91, 164
measuring 131, 156
percutaneous umbilical blood sampling (PUBS) *see* cordocentesis
perineum
damage to 33, 35, 203, 205
pain in 226, 231
see also episiotomy
tearing 33, 187, 202
pethidine 7, 59, 178, 187, 190-1, 215, 227
pinard 132, 180
placenta 30, 71, 121, 133, 148, 152, 153, 157, 172, 178, 195
delivery of 218-22
disposal of 222
inefficiency 166
pre-eclampsia 93
placenta praevia 100-101
caesarean section 211
post-mature pregnancy 166, 176
post-natal period 223-34
pain after caesarean 210
post-partum haemorrhage 19, 71, 73, 211
and birth chair 33
delivery of the placenta 220
forceps/ventouse and 226
'power struggles' 44-8
pre-eclampsia 80, 92-7, 98
early detection of 79
and elective caesarean 211
Pre-eclamptic Toxaemia Society 95, 97
pre-term labour/delivery 117, 221
and episiotomy 202
and pre-eclampsia 93, 96
brought on by smoking 101
and twins 87

pregnancy
confirming 127
difficulties during 78
privacy
in labour 15, 23-34
private hospitals 8-10
private midwives *see* independent midwives
prostaglandin
natural 169
synthetic 149, 168, 171-2, 178
protein
in urine 93, 129
pudendal block 194
pushing 28, 185, 201, 202, 208

respiratory depression 192
respiratory distress syndrome (RDS) 151
rhesus status 127-8
and fetomaternal haemorrhage 153
risk factors 146
Roberts, Helen 45
Robertson, Andrea 121
Royal College of Midwives 23, 24
Royal College of Obstetricians and Gynaecologists 40, 50, 61
rubella 77, 128

6-48 hour discharge 10, 13
scalp electrode 179, 182, 184-6
scan *see* ultrasound
screening tests 125, 126-41
see also individual tests
second opinion 73
and AFP test 144
and caesareans 216
and fetal distress 179
and ultrasound 138
semi-recumbent position 30, 202
senior house officer (SHO) 48, 64

sex
  after birth 203–4
  loss of interest 230–33
sexuality
  and birth 2, 122
sickness benefit 247
Simkin, Penny 225
six week check-up 224–8, 230
'smart cards' 119
smoking 78, 80, 101–3
social fund 252
Society and College of
  Radiographers 134
sonic aid *see* doppler
Spina Bifida 83, 127, 143,
  147, 150, 152, 158, 159
spinal block 193
squatting
  for breech delivery 90
  to avoid forceps delivery 207
  in labour 31–2, 168, 207
statutory maternity pay 246,
  247, 250–51
statutory sick pay 247, 252
stethoscope 132, 180
stillbirth 117
  caused by smoking 99, 101
stress
  caused by amniocentesis 147
  during ante-natal care 79, 80
  in labour 180
  caused by monitoring 180
  and pre-eclampsia 94
  smoking for 102
students 69–72
sudden infant death
  syndrome (SIDS)
  and smoking, 101
Support After Termination
  for Fetal Abnormality
  (SAFTA) 84
sweeping the membranes 175–7
syntocinon 28, 165, 171,
  172–3, 195, 220
syntometrine 219, 220

TENS 188
teaching hospitals 3
telemetry 186
television
  images of birth 29
termination 77, 79, 126,
  138, 144, 149
tests
  deciding about 157–9
Tew, Marjorie 62, 80
third stage of labour 218–22
tocolytics 89, 96, 162
tranquillisers
  for depression 229
  for pain 187, 191
  used with pethidine 191
  and pre-eclampsia 96
transvaginal ultrasound 134
transverse lie 91
twins 71, 87–9, 93, 150, 192
Twins and Multiple Births
  Association (TAMBA) 88

UKCC 65
  complaints to 239
  position on water birth 38
ultrasound 132–41, 180, 182
  use in amniocentesis 148
  breech baby 90
  use in cordocentesis 157
  use in CVS 153
  estimating delivery dates 115
  growth retardation 86
umbilical cord
  clamping 219
urine
  protein in 93, 129
  testing 129
uristix 129
'uterine hysteria' 162
uterine scar rupture
  with induction 173
  during VBAC 213
uterus 162, 164, 169, 178
  monitoring 195
  over-stimulation 172, 195, 201

rupture of non-scarred
  uterus 175

vacuum extraction 109, 201,
  205–9
  resulting in post-partum
  haemorrhage 226
vaginal birth after caesarean
  (VBAC) 212–13
  dangers of induction 172
vaginal examination 72, 131
vaginal prolapse 203
ventouse *see* vacuum
  extraction
violence
  technological 163
vomiting
  in labour 13–14
  during general
  anaesthetic 193

Wagner, Marsden 44
walking
  to augment labour 168
  during labour 28–30
water birth/labour 2, 34–8
water retention *see* oedema
weight gain 95, 99, 150
  ante-natal checks 130
  fear of getting fat 106
'white coat hypertension' 130
Who's Having Your Baby? 240
Women's Bodies, Women's Wisdom xiii
World Health Organisation
  xiii, 44
working
  after birth 254, 259

x-rays 137, 155

Yates, Paula 27–8
yoga 32, 110, 188

Of further interest...

Birth Tides

Turning towards Home Birth
Marie O'Connor

What is it really like to have a baby at home?

Many of us are familiar with the 'theory' of the revolt against hospitalized birth – but as more and more women around the world opt for home birth, what is the reality?

Marie O'Connor's groundbreaking and highly readable book is based on the real experiences of over 100 women who chose to give birth at home. Here are the true stories of painless natural birth – and of hard labours. Of babies coming out by themselves – and of babies who never want to come. Of unattended births – and of midwives who lift the pain away. Of absent fathers – and of partners acting as midwives, by accident and by design.

The poignant stories in *Birth Tides* are set against a worldwide trend towards 'actively' managing the 'patient' in labour; in the United States, one baby in four is born by Caesarean section. The author sees statistics such as this as the endpoint in a spiral of obstetrics in litigation. Good births, argues O'Connor, must involve autonomy for women, and this will require major changes in childbirth practices.

The Politics of Breastfeeding

Gabrielle Palmer

In a fully revised and updated new edition, this powerful and provocative book proves that breastfeeding is much more than a matter of personal inclination. Women all over the world are still being tricked into feeding their babies artificially and this affects us all: our health, our environment and the global economy.

Gabrielle Palmer asks whether bottlefeeding really does free women to lead more fulfilling lives. She examines social attitudes in a world where a woman who does breastfeed her child risks losing what little income she earns, and alerts us to the commercial reasons behind doctor's recommendations. With an engaging blend of facts, insight and anecdote, Gabrielle Palmer puts infant feeding 'fashions' into their historic and economic contexts. She shows how both poor and rich women suffer the consequences when men assume control over their bodies. She discusses the ecological effects of the decline in breastfeeding, the nutritional myths and the implications of such issues as radioactivity, breast cancer and AIDS.

The Tentative Pregnancy

Amniocentesis and the Sexual Politics of Motherhood
Barbara Katz Rothman

As more and more women are having children when they are over thirty, amniocentesis is becoming a routine part of prenatal care. In this groundbreaking book, Barbara Katz Rothman draws on the experience of over 120 women and a wealth of expert testimony to show how this simple procedure can radically alter the way we think about childbirth and parenthood. The results of amniocentesis, and the more recently developed chorion villus sampling, force us to confront agonizing dilemmas very early on: What do you do if there is a 'problem' with the fetus? What kind of support is available if you decide to raise a handicapped child? How can you come to terms with the termination of a wanted pregnancy?

Passionate, controversial and at times heartbreaking, *The Tentative Pregnancy* is a must for anyone thinking of having a child and for all those concerned with the growing proliferation of reproductive technology.

The Caesarean Experience

Dr Sarah Clement

In Britain around one in seven babies is born by caesarean section. Caesareans are an emotional and physical challenge, and this vital book provides all the information needed to have an informed discussion with your doctor.

Research psychologist and caesarean mother, Dr Sarah Clement, brings together the most up-to-date medical findings and over 200 women's caesarean experiences – both happy and difficult. Many vital but often neglected issues are addressed, including:

* the partner's emotions
* how to come to terms with a difficult caesarean experience
* how to have a Vaginal Birth After Caesarean (VBAC)

Every type of caesarean is covered: planned or emergency; with a general or epidural anaesthetic; with or without a partner present. Sarah Clement looks at the medical reasons for a caesarean section and offers practical advice for coping in the early weeks after the birth. She also shows how those caring for a caesarean mother can best support her before, during and after the birth, and suggests how women – and health professionals – can best avoid unnecessary caesarean sections and, when a caesarean is needed, ensure that it is a positive experience.

Drugs in Pregnancy and Childbirth

Judy Priest

This clear, practical guide will help every pregnant woman weigh up the risks and benefits of commonly prescribed and over-the-counter drugs, everyday things such as caffeine and alcohol, and the drugs which will probably be offered in labour.

A vitamin pill, an aspirin, a glass of wine, a cigarette with morning coffee or a doctor's prescription all take on new meaning when you are pregnant or trying to conceive. And when you are in labour, you will have to consider how the medication you might need will affect your baby.

Drawing on up-to-date research findings and women's real experiences and dilemmas, this book cuts through confusion and controversy to help you decide:

* which drugs, on balance, do more good than harm before conception, during pregnancy and while you are in labour
* what the consequences might be of taking or refusing a particular drug
* whether the drug might *benefit* your baby

And it will help you to live with your decisions.

This is a must for every woman who is concerned about her own welfare and her baby's health.

(Available from December 1996)

BIRTH TIDES	0 04 440916 8	£8.99	☐
THE POLITICS OF BREASTFEEDING	0 04 440877 3	£8.99	☐
THE TENTATIVE PREGNANCY	0 04 440912 5	£8.99	☐
THE CAESAREAN EXPERIENCE	0 04 440935 4	£7.99	☐
DRUGS IN PREGNANCY AND CHILDBIRTH	0 04 440492 1	£5.99	☐

All these books are available from your local bookseller or can be ordered direct from the publishers.

To order direct just tick the titles you want and fill in the form below:

Name: _____

Address: _____

_____

Postcode: _____

Send to Thorsons Mail Order, Dept 3, HarperCollins*Publishers*, Westerhill Road, Bishopbriggs, Glasgow G64 2QT.

Please enclose a cheque or postal order or your authority to debit your Visa/Access account –

Credit card no: _____

Expiry date: _____

Signature: _____

– up to the value of the cover price plus:

UK & BFPO: Add £1.00 for the first book and 25p for each additional book ordered.

Overseas orders including Eire: Please add £2.95 service charge. Books will be sent by surface mail but quotes for airmail dispatches will be given on request.

24-HOUR TELEPHONE ORDERING SERVICE FOR ACCESS/VISA CARDHOLDERS – TEL: 0141 772 2281.